The

Power, perseverance and
passion in lactation support

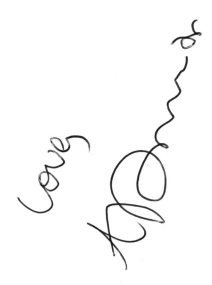

About the author

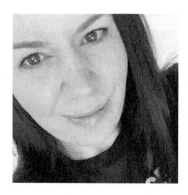

Amy Brown is a professor of public health based in the School of Health and Social Care at Swansea University in the UK. With a background in psychology, her research explores experiences of pregnancy, birth and early parenting with a particular focus on supporting infant feeding and mental health.

Amy is a respected international speaker and has published over 100 research papers, many of which underpin policy and practice guidelines including in the UK, Australia and USA. She is the author of twelve books including *Breastfeeding Uncovered* (2016; 2021), *Informed is Best* (2019) and *Covid Babies* (2021).

The Compassion Code

Power, perseverance and passion in lactation support

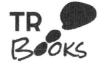

The Compassion Code: Power, perseverance and passion in lactation support

First published in the UK by Thought Rebellion Limited 2022

ISBN 978-1-7396929-1-9

Also available as an ebook

Proofread by Jules Wraith

Cover design: Leanne Pearce

A catalogue record for this book is available from the British Library.

Contents

Acknowledgements

As with any book there are many people I must thank who have played a role in its creation in one way or another. First, thank you to everyone who took part in the research study discussed in this book. Your eloquent responses helped spark the idea to write in depth about this subject and helped bring a challenging subject to life. I hope that it helps you reflect on a topic of huge importance and feel seen in the responses within this book.

Thank you also more broadly to all the parents, families, lactation supporters and healthcare professionals that I have worked alongside over the years (soon to be decades) as a breastfeeding and parenting researcher. Your stories and insights have helped stimulate research studies and thinking which I ultimately hope come back full circle to be of use and comfort to you.

Thank you also to my children who got me into this area of research in the first place. As teenagers now I'm sure you're delighted about me mentioning you here. Just remember though, my inclusion of you in other books allowed you to go to school on World Book days in your own clothes because you, as you quite rightly pointed out, were part of many books!

Thank you to Lyndsey Hookway for putting up with my 301 suggested titles for this book, stopping me from putting in too many references to my mid-life obsession with running and not rolling her eyes when I declared 'I actually think this book *might* be ok' (see chapter four for more discussion of our tendency towards impostor syndrome and doubting ourselves).

And finally thank you to my family and people who live in my phone messages who support me in every new crazy writing binge and life in general.

Introduction

I'm finishing this book in May 2022 during an unprecedented formula milk shortage in the USA. An inspection at an Abbott Nutrition owned plant in Michigan led to the discovery of Cronobacter sakazakii (formerly called Enterobacter sakazakii) in formula powder and on surfaces in the plant, halting production. Product shortages were then exacerbated by market domination of a small number of companies, strict import laws and supply chain issues.[1]

Of course, we know that another major contributor to this situation was a failure to invest in the needs of new families both through supporting breastfeeding and ensuring that infant formula supplies were not solely in the hands of a select industry. If governments valued breastfeeding and the health and wellbeing of mothers, babies and new parents through policies such as extended well-paid maternity leave, we may not have seen such a dire situation in the first place.

Why am I raising this issue? Because it is one of many infant feeding emergencies that is so central to the everyday experience of working in lactation support. Many lactation professionals and volunteers around the world have been watching the situation with dread, with some of you reading this book likely at the heart of it, working to support mothers, babies and families on the ground. Our hearts break for those families desperate to feed their babies, but our hearts also break for all the reasons we know led to this situation in the first place.

However, alongside this we are also dealing with the inevitable fall out in the media. On the one hand many are shouting about pressure to breastfeed and 'evil' lactation supporters supposedly hell bent on forcing breastfeeding upon everyone. On the other hand, unhelpful and seemingly malicious comments are made asking why women don't just breastfeed, blaming them for ending up in this situation as if it was somehow their fault.

As usual a core part of this appears to end up with lactation supporters being labelled as judgemental or failing to support all families. Of course, this could not be further from the truth. We support families through all sorts of feeding including when they cannot breastfeed. We support them through their grief at not being able to meet their feeding goals. We sit and listen to mothers' stories and strive to meet their needs, often against that backdrop of a complex system that doesn't value or understand breastfeeding, or experiences of mothering and caring for a baby. We leave at the end of the day, sometimes carrying the weight of their distress and sometimes buoyed by a success story. And yet media headlines continue to tell us that we're pressurising, or bullying, or only seeing infant feeding through one narrow (and judgemental) lens.

Sadly, this isn't an isolated event in the world of lactation support. We've been here before with similar crises whether that's through trying to fight unethical formula promotion tactics or supporting catastrophic events where poor care has devastatingly led to the harm or death of a baby. On a more day-to-day level many of us work in systems, whether that is healthcare, volunteering, or education, where we are seemingly the odd one out and considered anything from a slightly crazy maverick to an evangelical fool. Even when we feel fiercely supported by those around us, we are still fighting every day against a broader system of social injustice that does not value and invest in infant feeding in the way it deserves. So why carry on? Is this madness? Foolhardiness? Simple stubbornness at refusing to give in?

Possibly! But on a serious note, we carry on because this is not simply any old job or volunteering opportunity but a vocation that we are drawn to despite the barriers. It would be an injustice (and an exercise in mass deflation) to write this book simply focusing on the challenges of the role because the reality is that working in lactation support is so much more complex than that. In the same way that we find women in our care who are determined to breastfeed despite all the odds because breastfeeding is just so important to them, we continue in our roles because supporting them is just so important to us. As you will see throughout this book the challenges are undoubtedly real; but the joy, passion and satisfaction that many draw directly from the families that they support is even more so.

However, this does not mean that we need to be stoic martyrs who do not feel the complex emotions that working in this field brings. Recognising and naming those emotions, examining their antecedents and, more importantly, exploring ways in which we can also protect and care for ourselves in the same way we do for families in our care is vital. It not only ensures we maintain our own wellbeing but are also able to continue to care for families and fight systemic barriers in the future.

Unfortunately, we know from media headlines that high rates of stress and burnout are evident globally across healthcare professional fields with devastating impacts upon the rate at which staff are planning to leave their much loved occupation due to systems level factors such as understaffing, bullying and bureaucracy.[2] Indeed, research exploring the concepts of burnout and stress in midwifery, nursing and medical fields is increasingly well documented.[3,4] But on writing this book I was struck by how little research has explored the experiences of those caring for breastfeeding mothers and families.

Of course, some professionals working in midwifery and other healthcare roles will have lactation support as part of their job description. However, research exploring stress and burnout in healthcare professionals did not typically examine experiences of those supporting lactation and it left out the varied and valued experiences of everyone else working and volunteering in this field. Furthermore, as I will examine throughout this book, lactation support has its own specific challenges (and rewards) distinct from broader perinatal care. It is an important role in its own right and not simply a part of other perinatal health roles such as midwifery, health visiting and neonatal, or paediatric care.

Likewise, if you delve into the research literature you will now find lots of research about the complex challenges mothers and families face when it comes to breastfeeding and how these experiences can affect mental health. Indeed, some of my other books 'Breastfeeding Uncovered' and 'Why Breastfeeding Grief and Trauma Matter' explore this subject in depth. We know that breastfeeding is undermined by a system that does not value or support it and that experiences of battling this system can result in feelings of loss, grief and more.[5]

But it is not just parents who are affected by this – those working to support families within this system face the same challenges and have similar emotional scars. Yes, their experiences as professionals and volunteers will be different, but given that many in this field are brought here in the first place by their own feeding experiences, if anything this effect is multiplied.

We see the challenges of this broken system every day in our conversations with peers, in a battle to try to get something done, or being played out on social media. We know that we are fighting a system that doesn't properly value breastfeeding and a society that doesn't understand it. There is a seemingly never-ending tide of parents needing support. Arguments over pay - or the absence of it entirely. Frequent criticisms in the press, on social media and in-fighting sadly breaking out. The strange loneliness of the role especially when in the company of other professionals who don't support breastfeeding.

If we were to continue to look through just one lens, we would conclude that we are witnessing a profession under great strain, perhaps one that is haemorrhaging supporters every day. However, as you will see throughout this book, that would paint only part of the story and leaves out the passion and commitment that remains for many in the role. The rewards of seeing a family thrive. The sense of personal satisfaction and achievement. The thank you cards that make it all seem worthwhile a million times over. The stories of resilience and camaraderie. That baby who is breastfed despite all the odds. Or perhaps simply a drive to leave lactation support in a better place than where we first found it.

Who am I, and why is the wellbeing of lactation supporters so important to me?

For those of you who don't know me, I am a professor of maternal and child health at Swansea University in the UK where I lead the research centre Lactation, Infant Feeding and Translational research (LIFT). Although I trained as a peer supporter and then breastfeeding counsellor with the Association of Breastfeeding Mothers, my experience of supporting breastfeeding is now predominantly research-led, although I do spend considerable time on the battleground of social media sharing that work and talking to parents and those who support them. I have published over 100 research papers and books on infant feeding, many of which focus on the numerous complex psychological, social and cultural factors that affect decisions around breastfeeding and infant feeding.

My academic background is in psychology and since graduating, almost twenty years ago, I have had a particular interest in mental health and how it intertwines with feeding decisions and early parenting experiences. I have previously published widely on the mental health impacts of not being able to breastfeed, but a few years ago my experiences on social media and in talking to those working to support families on the ground led me to want to understand more about the mental health impacts of having a support role within this system.

I am all too aware of the pressures those working in lactation can experience through the stories (and shall we say 'challenging conversations') I see daily on my social media pages and the regular emails of despair and thanks (or sometimes anger) I receive from parents and those supporting them. Although I have experienced many positive encounters working with policy makers in my academic role, I've also had many soul-destroying ones where promises are not turned into action, or indeed the importance of breastfeeding from a physiological, relational and emotional perspective is simply dismissed. I understand the experience of having carefully crafted suggestions and plans ignored or trodden all over and having to watch the inevitable consequences of that play out in real people's lives.

The intertwine between infant feeding and mental health is central to my professional and personal life (which to be honest are a bit of a blur anyway - a theme you will see emerge later in this book). Like many of you reading this, the emotional load of this can weigh heavily, often fluctuating at speed from the joy of supporting a family to the utter frustration of seeing yet another mother let down. There is also a slight irony to all of this because 20 years ago I made the decision not to pursue my initial dream of qualifying as a clinical psychologist as I felt that trying to support trauma everyday would be really challenging. So I went into breastfeeding research instead. Maybe we just end up where we're meant to be (another core theme as you'll see in this book!).

Why is this book needed and where did it come from?

In 2019 (and then continuing through the early stages of the Covid-19 pandemic) I initially set out to conduct a research project exploring the issue of lactation supporters' wellbeing. I had been aware for a while that there was a gap in documented research in this area and was driven to start to fill it through many conversations with lactation supporters alongside having experienced some of the stressors of working in this arena myself. However, it was conducting the research for my book 'Why Breastfeeding Grief and Trauma Matter' that gave me the final push to start this research. It was strikingly clear to me that many of the emotions and experiences that women recounted in that book also applied to those working within the field (as indeed one survey respondent came to comment). Indeed, many of those writing about their own infant feeding experiences were now working in lactation support, precisely because of the long lasting impact of those experiences.

In part one of my research in 2019 I conducted a global survey exploring the wellbeing of those working across different lactation support roles. This was followed up by a shorter version during the Covid-19 pandemic in 2020 exploring how lockdown and changes to support may have affected lactation supporter wellbeing. Over 700 professionals and volunteers who were working to support breastfeeding responded to that initial research request, pouring their heart into describing the stresses of their role, what keeps them going and strategies for change. A further 520 took part in the Covid-19 questionnaire. Both surveys had ethics permission from my university research ethics committee.

What was striking in the results was the number of free text comments thanking me for doing this research alongside the richness and depth of the open-ended data. Although my initial intention was to simply publish an academic article, it was clear that the data was much more complex than that and intertwined with a lot of my work exploring societal influences upon infant feeding.

It was also clear that the work could be useful in both highlighting the issue of stress and burnout in the lactation field but also to serve as something productive to practically help support the wellbeing of those on the ground. Alongside identifying the stressors that you face and exploring and validating the logic of those feelings I also want this book to offer hope through three chapters: Why we carry on, Tools for support, and a Manifesto for change. I hope that on reading this book that you feel heard but also encouraged and supported.

What do I mean by the 'lactation profession'?

I use the terms 'lactation profession' and 'lactation supporters' throughout this book. During the creative and editing process for designing this book we thought long and hard about the best word to use that would capture its role and ethos. Lactation was chosen over terms such as infant feeding or breastfeeding because it is a globally used term. It mirrors wording used in committees and roles, such as lactation consultant, and felt like the word to use to describe the vocation of lactation work and support, thus separating it from a book about supporting breastfeeding. It is also a word that reflects the broader work of the role. Some families that you will be supporting have a baby who is not directly breastfed. They may be exclusively pumping; others may have a baby who is tube-fed, and donor milk may feature.

Whatever your role is, I want you to feel that this term includes everyone who works to support mothers and families with breastfeeding and the wider challenges of feeding their baby. This may be in a professional or voluntary capacity. You may have specific infant feeding qualifications or not. You may earn money in your role or not. But whatever your title or role, supporting breastfeeding is at the heart of what you do. You are part of the shared experience of wanting to protect breastfeeding and responsive parenting in a world that at best doesn't understand it, and at worst actively fights against it. I hope that this book will be relevant for:

- Healthcare and medical professionals
- Lactation consultants
- Breastfeeding counsellors and specialists
- Breastfeeding peer supporters
- Doulas and parent supporters
- Charity leads, Trustees, Milk banking staff and others
- Academics working in infant feeding research
- Advocates and those who support on social media

A quick note here. This book brings together data from lactation professionals and volunteers from around the world. Next to each quote in the book I have given an abbreviated description of the role the individual has and their country. If they are also a healthcare professional (*abbreviation HCP*) I have provided that detail. Terminology and preference of title are slightly different in different languages and countries (or even within countries depending on where people train).

For readability and comparison, I have used the term International Board Certified Lactation Consultant (*abbreviation IBCLC*) for anyone who has passed this exam. I have used the term Peer Supporter for those working in breastfeeding / mother to mother peer support groups. These individuals may have had very different levels of training, have different role remits, and some may be paid. Likewise, those using the term breastfeeding counsellor or breastfeeding specialist are likely to have had more intense training than those in peer support posts but less than those in lactation consultant posts.

Where an individual had more than one qualification I chose to use the likely more recent and current qualification in their quote description i.e. breastfeeding counsellor rather than peer supporter (otherwise some role descriptions would be longer than the quote!). My initial plan was to also add location to the quotes to show the breadth of response from a global perspective, for example 'IBCLC, UK'. However, on reflection we decided during the editing process that this risked speculation as to the identity of the respondent, especially in regions where there is a relatively small pool of any one professional group. Some respondents may have been happy with being potentially identifiable, but we did not want to take that risk. However, please be assured that the quotes used in this book are drawn from across participant locations, reflecting responses in North and South America, Australasia, the UK and Ireland, Europe, Southeast Asia, the Middle East, and South Africa.

Finally, as with my other books, this book takes an inclusive stance and recognises that you will be supporting families with many identities and preferred words for themselves and how they feed their baby including breastfeeding, human milk, lactation and chest feeding. It goes without saying that you may have your own preferred terms. Ease of reading unfortunately prevents inclusion of all terms throughout every reference to feeding babies in the book, but I fully recognise that some personally prefer not to use the word breast for reasons such as trauma whilst others feel strongly about using it. In short, I am conscious that there is no one way to write so that everyone will feel their needs are best met, and that discussions over this issue can divide opinion.

I have used additive language throughout the book, particularly in relation to mother, parent and families - although I frequently refer to breastfeeding parents and families as the plural because of the huge potential of them to influence feeding outcomes. We also *do* work with partners and families. However, the majority of the research that I cite is based on participants described as women and mothers so those are the terms I use most frequently. I have, of course, left all quotes from participants in the research as they were given, using the terminology and phrases they chose to use.

Who took part in the research used in this book?

Overall, 727 lactation professionals, healthcare professionals and volunteers took part in the first survey. Some key demographic statistics from the sample include:

- Age: The average age of people responding was 40 with a range from 18 – 73 years.

- Sex: 723 female, 1 male and 3 non-binary.

- Sexuality: 56 respondents identified as lesbian, bi-sexual, queer, asexual or gender fluid.

- Dependent children: 548 had children under the age of 18 living at home.

- Location: 546 lived in the UK with other respondents from the USA (n = 65), Europe (n = 40), Australia (n = 27), Southeast Asia (n = 14), Canada (n = 13), New Zealand (n = 12), Middle East (n = 5), South America (n = 3) and Africa (n = 2).

- Ethnicity: 72% of those who responded to this question described themselves as White (i.e. White British, White American, White European). Given the global nature of the survey it is complex to list every ethnicity given variations in personal identity and differences in phrasing between countries. However, some of the largest groups that responded included Mixed or multiple race (n = 68), Chinese (n = 19), Southeast Asian (n = 18), Jewish (n = 11), Black (n = 9) and Asian (n= 8).

In terms of roles, many participants wore many hats! As you can see from the list below the numbers do not add up to 100% for this reason. Overall:

- 21% had an IBCLC role / qualification
- 32% had a breastfeeding counsellor role / qualification
- 49% had a peer supporter role / qualification
- 18% had a health professional role
- 8% had a charity role not directly related to supporting mothers and families
- 4% had a doula role / qualification
- 3% had a maternity support worker role
- 20% were breastfeeding advocates on social media
- 4% were tongue tie specialists

A further 13% had 'other' roles including research, postnatal support, antenatal breastfeeding educators, author, board members of charities/CIC, trainees for peer support, counselling or IBCLC roles, policy advisors, childbirth educators and complementary therapists.

Health professionals who completed the survey predominantly noted that they were midwives, health visitors, maternity support workers and child/ family nurses. Several doctors, including general practitioners (GPs), neonatal and paediatric specialists took part. One participant noted that they worked in an emergency unit in a general role but were often called upon if a mother came to the unit with 'feeding issues'. Another participant had a broader role within a children's centre but often gave support to breastfeeding mothers. One dentist also responded, predominantly in her role as a peer supporter, but adding in further experience from her dentistry role. As an aside, this really does show the value of making sure all roles who encounter new families have ample opportunity for breastfeeding specific training as some may be influencing parents without having the knowledge and experience of those in the survey.

The sample was varied in how long participants had been working in lactation support. Around a third had two years' experience or less and half had over ten years. The prize for the longest service went to a participant with 47 years' service although she was in good company as 8% of the sample had over 25 years' experience.

In terms of where participants gave support, 48% conducted home visits, 26% worked in specialist clinics, 67% were involved with peer support groups, 48% in a hospital setting, 17% did some work in an office, 44% gave phone call support, 39% email support, 47% text support, 36% other messaging support such as WhatsApp, and 62% provide support via social media. Other settings listed included antenatal groups, tongue tie clinics, emergency wards, children's centres, church, and pregnancy yoga. Really, anywhere where families attended or as one respondent noted *'In the most random places – school gate, family events, supermarket, playground etc'*.

In part two of the study which was conducted during Covid-19, 520 people took part. The average age was 38 with a range from 22 - 71 years. Overall, 518 were female and two non-binary. Twenty-eight identified as lesbian, bisexual or queer. In terms of dependent children, 402 had children under the age of 18 living at home. For ethnicity, 390 described themselves as White with some of the other largest groups including mixed or multiple race (n = 67), Chinese (n = 22), Southeast Asian (n = 17), Black (n = 9), Asian (n = 6), and Jewish (n = 5). For location, 392 lived in the UK with further responses from USA (n = 43), Australia (n = 24), Europe (n = 23), Southeast Asia (n = 13), Canada (n = 10), New Zealand (n = 10), Middle East (n = 3), and South America (n = 2).

Again, professional roles were varied with some holding multiple roles. Overall:

- 33% had an IBCLC role
- 29% had a breastfeeding counsellor role
- 65% had a peer supporter role (44% as sole role)
- 5% had a charity role not directly related to supporting mothers and families
- 3% had a doula role
- 28% had a health professional role
- 4% had a maternity support worker role
- 25% were breastfeeding advocates on social media
- 2% were tongue tie specialists

A further 19% again had 'other' roles including academia/research, postnatal support, antenatal breastfeeding educators, author, board members of charities/CIC, trainees for peer support, counselling or IBCLC roles, policy advisors, childbirth educators and complementary therapists.

With my research geek hat on this sample, like any research, has its limitations. It is likely that those most concerned about their wellbeing and who perhaps had experienced the most challenges were more motivated to take part. The survey was also shared via social media. The benefits of this include the global reach as seen in the survey demographics but do limit likely participation to those active on social media (although some participants noted that they shared the survey with colleagues who were not on social media groups).

Another limitation is that the survey focused mainly on the challenging aspects of the lactation role, and how to improve these. It was designed to measure burnout and different stressors, alongside exploring the positives and strategies for strength and resilience. It was not designed to measure all positive aspects of the role, although it definitely does draw on the positives and silver linings. What it certainly isn't without is hope. The hope and vision for a positive future clearly shone out through participants' responses, despite recognising the significant challenges of their roles.

Finally, as an unfunded study, participation was limited to those who could complete it in the English language which also reduced accessibility. The survey included few respondents from the global south, presenting a picture predominantly of those working in more affluent regions but where breastfeeding rates are typically lower from a global perspective. This response really shows the need for a larger collaborative survey that ensures greater representation and global diversity.

Why the 'Compassion Code'?

During the creative and editing process for this book we thought long and hard about what to call this book. Seriously, sometimes coming up with a book title is harder than writing the actual book in the first place! We settled on the word compassion after reflecting on all the findings in the survey and the broader literature around lactation and breastfeeding support. When trying to think of 'words that sum up the book' the word compassion stood out.

Compassion is at the heart of what we do in lactation support and is often what keeps us going through all the challenges. But it's also what we need to give more of to ourselves. One of the lines I will repeat several times in this book is the hope that on reading this you treat yourself with the same kindness and compassion that you show the women, parents and families that you care for.

The subtitle came from the strengths that drive many of us forward (and we do also love a bit of alliteration). What we didn't want was this to be a negative book that focussed on the challenges of the role alone. These clearly need identifying and reflecting on, but what was clear throughout survey responses was that there is another side - a draw that brings you back day after day to keep on keeping on. There is indeed such power, perseverance and passion in those who support breastfeeding, lactation and families - and that's what we wanted to focus on.

What do I want you to do with this book?

Ultimately, I hope that reading this book will leave you in a better place where you can:

- Feel validated and 'seen' in the shared responses and reflections of others in the lactation field

- Reflect on the challenges that come with your role and how they can lead to feelings of frustration, burnout and compassion fatigue

- Separate feelings of frustration and fatigue at broader systemic challenges away from the experience of working day to day with families in the community

- Feel motivated by the 'reasons to keep on carrying on' and recognise the balance in the challenges and rewards in your role

- Develop new strategies for supporting your own wellbeing and those that you work alongside

- Continue with the fight for a better future for us all

Chapter 1

The rollercoaster of joy and burnout in the lactation field

Lactation support is an incredibly rewarding role but one that I know comes with significant pressures, challenges and responsibilities. As highlighted in the introduction, understanding how professionals and volunteers working in this field are feeling and what support they need to grow and develop in their roles is vital for many reasons. It is of course important for those giving the support. But we also know that high quality and timely lactation support plays a vital role in enabling women to breastfeed for longer.[1] Without that support where would families be? What would our communities look like? Our future?

The vital importance of the role means that we need to value and support the mental health of those who work in lactation for everyone's sake - the families, those who support them, and the families of the future. However, in a role seemingly filled with a never-ending stream of parents needing support and the challenges of the work, it is easy to forget to care for ourselves too. In urging you to think about your own wellbeing I am asking you to do the work-based equivalent of putting your own oxygen mask on before trying to help others.

Although there is a dearth of research exploring the mental health of those working in lactation support, we can learn a lot from research that has explored the wellbeing of healthcare professionals in other roles. If we look to related fields of nursing, midwifery, health visiting, and medicine, the emotional intensity of roles that involve closely working with families is well recognised.

For example, Professor Billie Hunter has talked extensively about the *'emotion work'* that many midwives must undertake in their everyday role, supporting families through their anxieties and stressors.[2] Likewise, emotion work is a major part of the health visiting role with compassion and understanding vital to caring for and supporting families through experiences such as postnatal depression and birth trauma.[3]

Emotion work is often a valued part of many healthcare professionals' roles and is in part what motivates many to train and practice. Unfortunately, the importance and intensity of this work is often not felt to be recognised or valued by those in higher management roles.[4] Moreover, the intensity of providing emotional support to families and the strain this can place on a practitioner's wellbeing is recognised across healthcare professions including nurses, general practitioners, paediatricians and other medical roles. The impact of this work has been strongly linked to risk of burnout especially if little support and opportunity for a break is provided.[5]

On top of this, there is increasing recognition in research, reports and news headlines that healthcare professionals are working in a world of escalating institutional and societal pressures and barriers.[6] Recently the staffing crisis and pressure on midwives has reached the news, although burnout and frustrations are also at boiling point amongst many other healthcare roles.[7]

Examining the research and stories behind the midwifery burnout headlines we can see that aspects of the role unrelated to what drew many to it in the first place are often to blame. For example, staffing shortages and underfunding, a lack of understanding about the value of their role, bullying and bureaucracy are all closely tied to burnout and disillusionment.[8]

This stress is multiplying over the years coupled with increasing political and public debate around 'normality' and interventions during childbirth.[9] Many fear that they cannot safely care for women, or care for them in the way they have been trained, with over half saying they wanted to leave the profession in the next year. It is worrying that almost all who had been working in the NHS for five years or less did not feel valued by the government.[10]

Likewise, the Institute of Health Visiting has raised the alarm over staffing crises and the wellbeing of their workforce. Even before the Covid-19 pandemic, drastic budget cuts in recent years have left health visitors concerned for the safety of the families that they care for, worried that impossibly high caseloads mean that they will miss signs of something being wrong, or not able to offer families all the support that they need.

Between 2015 and 2019 almost one in five health visiting posts was lost, with almost half of health visitors stating that they were so worried about understaffing that they feared a tragedy would occur. Many spent their days feeling tense and anxious, with some describing how they have had to numb themselves to the plight of families in their caseload as it is simply too much to bear.[11]

This issue only increased during the Covid-19 pandemic with many health visitors redeployed to other roles meaning that while the needs of many vulnerable families grew during lockdowns, the number of health visitors able to support them diminished. I will return to this later in the book but as you might expect this had a devastating impact upon the mental health and wellbeing of health visitors with many feeling that they were no longer delivering a quality service and failing the families they were meant to be serving.[12]

Indeed, many working in healthcare are facing these pressures. For example, the General Medical Council in the UK recently released a report showing that burnout amongst trainee doctors and trainers was at the highest levels since measurements began in 2018 with three in five reporting they always or often felt worn out at the end of a working day, and 44% stating that their work was 'emotionally exhausting' to a high or very high degree.[13]

This report is not alone - a survey by the British Medical Council found that a third of medics are suffering from burnout and compassion fatigue, with A&E doctors and GPs having the highest levels.[14] Again, the trauma experienced during the course of their job, long working hours and increasing patient numbers to support are at the heart of this.[15] Does all of this sound rather too familiar?

Experiences of supporting breastfeeding

So how do the experiences of those working in lactation support fit into this pattern? On an experiential and anecdotal level I could write a book on this alone. But even if we look for research exploring the broader experiences of supporting breastfeeding, there is surprisingly little published on the motivations, wellbeing and experiences of those working in lactation support. Countless papers have examined families' experiences of breastfeeding support, but often, to find evidence of experience of being a lactation supporter you have to dig into papers examining maternal experiences where sometimes you might find a line or two about the supporters.

So what *has* been published on this topic? Well, to start with the positives; providing breastfeeding support can feel incredibly empowering, especially if it results in an improved infant feeding experience for a mother.[16] It can be a rewarding social experience, connecting with like-minded others and feeling part of a supportive community.[17] It can provide significant personal reward and joy, feeling like you are doing something positive with your time, helping families and communities, and contributing to a better society.[18]

This intrinsic motivation to make a difference is a vital part of interventions that are put in place to help improve breastfeeding. Without the motivation and support of those who deliver breastfeeding support, strategies are likely to fail.[19] When I looked at open ended survey responses, this depth and breadth of emotion was clear to see - many lactation supporters simply loved their role and took great pleasure and joy in it.

'I love what I do and being able to give back and support families. I can't imagine me without it.' (Peer supporter)

One of the most common words used within the survey was 'reward'. Many felt that the role brought them great personal reward and delighted at being able to take play a role in supporting families.

> 'Breastfeeding support is one of the hardest jobs I've done but the most rewarding.' (Breastfeeding counsellor)

> 'It is exhausting but so rewarding.' (IBCLC)

Central to this were feelings of privilege of being able to be in such a position. Supporters were proud of their role and identity and the work that they did, thriving in their role and feeling lucky at being able to support others:

> 'I love peer supporting. I feel very lucky to be in a face-to-face voluntary role.' (Peer supporter)

> 'It is an absolute privilege to be able to serve families in this role.' (IBCLC)

Another core feeling was that of empowerment. Many talked about how the work, although frustrating at times, brought a great sense of accomplishment when they were able to support and improve things for a family. This reaction was most frequently raised by peer supporters:

> 'I couldn't imagine not giving support. It's really empowering although sometimes it's just a never-ending battle against misinformation and other professionals.' (Peer supporter)

> 'I absolutely love my role and I think there is something so empowering about women helping women, even if it does sometimes feel like the wider healthcare system/ government doesn't value what we do.' (Peer supporter)

There was also a feeling of relief and gratitude at being able to serve in such a role when a supporter had themselves received good support or overcome a difficult infant feeding journey:

'I feel that I am giving back to those who once supported me all those years ago.' (IBCLC)

'Replenishing the system with what I took is important to me.' (Breastfeeding counsellor)

The word 'responsibility' emerged many times across responses. Although some days this responsibility could weigh heavily, at its core was a feeling of duty to use knowledge and skills to help others. Some described it as a calling, whereas others felt that their natural skills and passionate interest brought them to the work. In communities where breastfeeding was underfunded and undervalued, the importance of showing up to support families and the satisfaction this brought was clear.

'I have a responsibility now to help others with the knowledge I have accumulated. Even if I wanted to, I couldn't walk away.' (IBCLC)

'I feel a deep responsibility to the families that I work with. It may be hard at times but it's what I feel I am designed to do.' (Peer supporter)

However, although there are strong motivators for working in lactation support, many professionals and volunteers painted a much more nuanced and mixed picture of their experiences. In the survey participants were asked how often they felt a range of different emotions relating to their day-to-day role. What emerged was a very interesting pattern.

Overall, frustration, exhaustion and other negative emotions were common but simultaneously many felt high levels of satisfaction and reward. For example, over 75% of supporters described 'often' feeling 'frustrated', 'helpless' and 'undermined'. But at the same time, a similar proportion reported feeling 'rewarded', 'satisfied I've done a good job' and 'privileged to be in this role'.

Other emotions such as 'valued' were more mixed and open-ended responses suggested this was context dependent and varied between situations. Sometimes it was possible to feel competing emotions at the same time, or at least in quick succession depending on who you were interacting with. I will return to this later but as one infant feeding lead explained:

> *'Some days it feels like a rollercoaster. You're pulling your hair out because you can't organise a room for the peer supporters to run a group or have heard that yet another mother has been given incorrect advice by another professional. But then you get a thank you card from a grateful family or see the difference in someone's face when they finally latch their baby on pain free. Some days, when my husband asks me 'how was work' I genuinely do not know what to say or where to begin.' (Infant feeding lead)*

This concurrent mixture of both positive and negative emotions is interesting. You might expect that consistent strong negative emotions and experiences would leave people feeling downtrodden and exhausted – and ready to leave their roles. However, it really did seem that although many were under immense stress, the positives of the role somehow overrode this (or at least they did once you'd had a chance to decompress and reflect).

Notably, as I will explore further throughout this book, a key safety net to the high stress that many respondents felt was that emotions appeared to be ring-fenced or compartmentalised. A typical experience of a practitioner or volunteer was significant frustration with 'the system' coupled with considerable reward from being able to help families and feel like they were making a difference. These two competing experiences appeared to exist separately rather than affecting each other. No matter how high the frustration it didn't mean that the core role of helping families was ruined:

> *'I hate the paperwork and nonsense but I love the families. It kinda evens itself out.' (Midwife)*

> *'I've been broken by colleagues who should know better but even in my darkest moments I'm buoyed back up by the gratitude of families.' (IBCLC)*

To sum up, it was clear from responses in the survey that lactation support was certainly not a boring or 'numb' role for many to say the least. It elicited many emotions on a day-to-day basis and those working across the field certainly felt an emotional reaction to the work that they did. There's something here about feeling that the role certainly reminds you that you are alive - boredom is one word that was never used in the survey! But what happens when those emotions become too much?

When things get more serious – burnout and compassion fatigue

Although many working in lactation support and other caring professions will recognise the day-to-day stress and strain of the role, it is important to distinguish between a normal reaction to a challenging role that goes away after a break or when things ease (or indeed after a long rant with trusted colleagues), and more long-lasting signs of stress, anxiety or depression, and burnout. Spotting the signs of when something is becoming overwhelming is a really important part of affording yourself the same level of care that you afford others every day - but is something that many of us drawn to the world of lactation support often find very difficult to do.

Sadly, we know that mental health challenges are all too common in healthcare related roles. In a recent study of UK midwives, over a third were displaying moderate to high symptoms of stress, anxiety and depression and this was more common in younger midwives or those with fewer than ten years' experience.[20] Rates were slightly lower at around 20% in a similar Australian study,[21] but that still represents a rate of one in five midwives struggling with their mental health.

Some studies suggest an even higher prevalence rate for nursing staff, with an Australian study finding a third to a half of nurses showing clinical signs of depression, stress or anxiety,[22] with similar rates found in studies in Hong Kong[23] and the USA.[24] Likewise, research with medical students and medical professionals highlights that in some studies up to two thirds are showing clinical levels of anxiety and depression, although many studies point to around a third - which, of course, is still too high.[25] As you might expect, many of these rates have increased across professional groups on a global level during the Covid-19 pandemic due to unprecedented pressures around workload, staffing and safety.[26]

Turning to the concept of burnout, this issue presents another serious challenge for those working in healthcare professions. The concept of burnout was first identified by Freudenberger, who was a German-born American psychologist. It has attracted considerable research attention over the years by psychologists, but some of the most famous work has been conducted by Christina Maslach and Susan Jackson who identified three core elements of this syndrome: exhaustion, depersonalisation and hopeless and cynical feelings around personal accomplishment.[27]

In recent years burnout has been added to the International Classification of Diseases (ICD) which is a diagnostic tool that looks at disease and health outcomes. The International Classification of Diseases 11th revision (published in 2019) describes burnout as *'A syndrome conceptualised as resulting from chronic workplace stress that has not been successfully managed'.*[28] The ICD-11 considers burnout to have three core factors:

- Feelings of energy depletion or exhaustion
- Increased mental distance from one's job, or feelings of negativism or cynicism related to one's job
- Reduced professional efficacy

The ICD emphasises that burnout is an occupational phenomenon – something that stems from your job experience rather than being a medical or mental health condition in its own right. In other words, burnout doesn't stem from you, it stems from the pressures of your job. If you didn't have your job, you wouldn't be burnt out. Burnout risk is clearly linked to occupational stress including working long hours, a lack of control over your role and outcomes, and continually dealing with situations that are high stress.[29] It really is not you – it's them! Although many solutions focus on building resilience in the individual, what really should be happening is a change to working conditions so that such high resilience was not needed in the first place.

When stress and exhaustion turn to burnout the results are often catastrophic. The person who once was passionate and loved their work can become detached and bitter.[30] As you can imagine, burnout is associated with a whole host of negative health outcomes including insomnia, anxiety and depression, relationship difficulties and substance misuse.[31,32] It can result in healthcare professionals leaving their roles, or starting to experience significant compassion fatigue (more on this later).[33]

Guilt is another common reaction. Research with midwives who have experienced burnout finds that many feel full of guilt and self-blame at not being able to 'cope' with the demands of their role. Even though it is the stressors and demands of the system that have understandably led to exhaustion, many still felt like failures rather than seeing that the system had failed them.[34] There is a clear overlap here between how many women who have not been able to breastfeed feel, carrying the blame and thinking they were not good enough, when in fact it was the system who failed them.[35]

As introduced above, compassion fatigue is closely related to burnout. Compassion fatigue occurs when previously very motivated healthcare professionals start to care less and less about the families they are working with. First identified in nurses working in emergency care in 1992, considerable research has since explored this phenomenon.[36] A central part of compassion fatigue is struggling to feel any empathy or compassion for others - which as you likely know are vitally important aspects of caring work. What essentially happens is that due to sustained and intolerable levels of stress and pressure, professionals can no longer cope with feeling such intense levels of emotion, become desensitised and shut down.

Many consider compassion fatigue to be a physiological response to high levels of continued stress rather than simply a reaction to the emotional pressures of caring roles. The demands of many healthcare roles such as long working hours, exposure to traumatic situations and the importance of decisions made, mean that stress levels are often raised in the body. Levels of stress hormones such as adrenaline and corticosterone rise in response to stressful work situations, which cause physiological symptoms as part of the fight or flight stress response, such as increasing heart rate and blood pressure.

This response was designed to allow us to deal with stressful situations quickly by fighting or running away. It was never designed to be a long-term response. However, the demands of healthcare roles mean that there is little opportunity for 'escape' (and fighting is not recommended), which keeps stress hormones and the associated response high. We know that this sustained stress response is linked to reduced immune function, increased levels of obesity, cardiovascular disease and mental health issues.[37]

Compassion fatigue has been viewed as the eventual collapse of this stress response - i.e. we cannot simply continue running at that level of stress forever. Many consider it to be a protective mechanism in some way, allowing the individual to escape from the sustained stress that they are under. They have not been able to 'fight' or 'flee' from the stressful situation so to protect the body, the third option is to stop considering the situation stressful.

A central part of our body's physiological stress response is labelling a situation as stressful and therefore in lieu of being able to deal with the stress in other ways, the brain makes a cognitive decision to not be bothered by the stressors in front of it. This means that you can lose the feelings of stress but also subsequently lose feelings of empathy and passion. As two professionals described:

'I have become hardened over my many years of service and don't respond in the same way anymore. I do still care but I certainly don't feel it as vividly and deeply as I did back at the start of my nursing career.' (Health visitor)

'I used to get angry at injustice but these days I often feel numb. I wonder if this is the consequence of seeing the same problems over and over. You can't react with anger forever.' (IBCLC)

Others have described compassion fatigue as a trauma response, with healthcare professionals blocking out and trying to avoid memories of their trauma (or in other words their everyday work). Trauma can occur when we ourselves feel that our life or wellbeing is put at risk, or we witness others have an accident or lose their life. The continual witnessing of others having accidents or experiencing traumatic events that threaten their health or wellbeing (including poor care) becomes overwhelming.

To protect itself from the emotional trauma the brain shuts off its emotional response.[38]

Trauma often presents with difficulty eating or sleeping, hypervigilance and being on edge, concentration issues and anger - all of which are classic symptoms of burnout. Indeed, this trauma response was clear amongst survey responses with many feeling traumatised by seeing such high levels of poor care and overwhelming grief in those they were supporting:

> *'Seeing the suffering of mothers at the hands of others can feel all too much.' (Breastfeeding counsellor)*

> *'I feel traumatised by the trauma of the many mothers I see.' (IBCLC)*

Compassion fatigue has also been linked to an intense need of many healthcare professionals to want to improve the lives of the patients and families they care for. When they are repeatedly not able to do this, often through no fault of their own, they experience intense guilt and as a consequence shut off from those that they are caring for.[39] It is not that they have run out of compassion but simply that they cannot bear to feel the weight of not being able to save those they care for, even when it is not directly their fault or within their power to save them.

This is likely a core element of burnout and compassion fatigue for many in the lactation field. Some days the continual tide of external pressures from a lack of government funding, exploitative industry and unhelpful societal messaging just feels too strong. Indeed, guilt was evident in many survey responses:

> *'Many nights, reflecting on the long day, I feel such guilt for those I could not help.' (IBCLC)*

> *'Nothing prepares you for the guilt of not being able to help a mother.' (Peer supporter)*

A final proposal for the causes of compassion fatigue is simple frustration at those that you are caring for not heeding advice or taking care of themselves. For example, a doctor may become frustrated at a patient who repeatedly fails to take advice or make any changes to behaviours that are having a significant, detrimental impact upon their illness. As a result, they become despairing, shutting down from caring because they think that there is no point.[40]

In survey responses this reaction was not present directly in relation to those who were trying to overcome breastfeeding challenges but was clearly identifiable in relation to broader societal influences. Some observed, at least some days, that trying to support breastfeeding in a society that doesn't value or understand it felt like a phenomenal waste of time:

'I do have moments sometimes where I think this is a pointless career. What difference can I make against all those who wish to undermine breastfeeding? It would seem easier not to care.' (IBCLC)

'Sometimes I feel ineffectual in my role supporting other people who are supporting breastfeeding women. They feel powerless to change things for the better, and I in turn feel powerless to help them change things because of wider societal problems that can't be solved.' (Breastfeeding counsellor, Charity role)

Alongside the reduction in empathy experienced, those suffering from compassion fatigue may experience many physiological symptoms such as headaches, insomnia, feeling exhausted, and other physical health symptoms. Feelings of irritability, anxiety, depression, cynicism and hopelessness are common. At a personal level compassion fatigue is linked to relationship difficulties, substance misuse and mental health issues. On a work level those experiencing compassion fatigue are more likely to make poor clinical decisions, be absent from work and of course, ultimately leave their position.[41]

One interesting element of compassion fatigue, that I feel is notable, is the finding that those experiencing it may adopt what has been termed a 'silencing response' to individuals that they are caring for who are expressing emotions or talking about their trauma. For example, they shut down a cancer survivor from talking about their illness or dismiss it as not mattering because they survived their treatment.[42]

How often do we hear from those we care for that they were told by a healthcare professional that their breastfeeding experience is irrelevant or not important? How many women are dismissed and told to simply give formula without any consideration of how they might be feeling? Although we know that this is a broader issue around how society views breastfeeding and human milk, might some of this be linked to compassion fatigue? It is certainly a lens through which to reflect when we are feeling frustrated at poor support being provided to families. How far would supporting healthcare professionals to debrief their own infant feeding experiences take us?

Thousands of papers have now been published on the risk factors, occurrence and impacts of compassion fatigue across the healthcare professions including midwives, nurses, doctors, paramedics and allied health professionals. Many published studies find that globally, over half of their sample are at moderate to high risk of compassion fatigue above levels of work-related burnout.[20,43,44] Research is starting to document how other perinatal health professionals such as doulas and maternity support workers are also experiencing burnout although it is still sparse at present.[45]

Notably, just as with burnout, those at the start of their careers who are being exposed to stressors for the first time are at a higher risk of compassion fatigue. Additionally, female health care professionals are typically at a much higher risk than male. It has been hypothesised that this is due to wider structural factors including being more likely to have to balance work alongside other caring responsibilities, still taking on the majority of household chores and sexism in the workplace making it harder to progress, earn a higher salary and be respected.[46] One study found that women in the workplace had less autonomy and authority leaving them feeling frustrated, overburdened and with less control over their work.[47]

Other studies have pinpointed a higher level of impostor syndrome in women as a key factor (which we will return to in chapter four).[48] Finally, female healthcare professionals are at a greater risk of clinical anxiety and depression than men, which likely increases risk.[49]

Risk factors for compassion fatigue include all those you might expect - too many hours, too many patients, too much bureaucracy, too many high risk situations.[50] One that I felt was particularly relevant to the lactation profession, and will come back to later, identified the blurring of personal and professional boundaries as a risk.[51] When professionals struggled to maintain boundaries between their personal and professional lives, continually worked longer hours than they should and regularly took problems home with them, their risk of burnout was greater. Does this remind you of anyone?

Burnout in the lactation profession

Turning our attention to burnout and compassion fatigue in the lactation profession, there is very little recognition of this issue in the literature. Again, although health care professionals who have lactation support as part of their role may be experiencing burnout symptoms related to infant feeding support, this has not been explicitly measured, nor in other lactation support roles.

The importance of the issue has however been highlighted numerous times. In 2013 Dr Kathy Kendall-Tackett, as editor in chief of the journal Clinical Lactation, raised this issue in her editorial column highlighting its occurrence in the lactation field.[52] There have been a several excellent talks considering how to manage burnout and compassion fatigue following this, including ones by Dr Kendall-Tackett, Nekisha Killings, Kathy Parkes and Leah Jolly and Annie Frisbie (for details of how to access these see the last chapter on further resources).

However, in terms of published research studies there was nothing I could find that specifically tackled mental health in relation to breastfeeding support. As previously noted, research has explored stress, burnout and compassion fatigue within midwifery, nursing, medicine and neonatal care but a search through hundreds of these papers found nothing explicitly related to the experience of supporting lactation.

This is despite a clear need and recognition of the ramifications for the profession. Concern for this growing issue, specifically in relation to the Covid-19 pandemic, was highlighted in an editorial feature in the Journal of Human Lactation in 2022.[53] Likewise, anecdotal reflections on witnessing increasing signs of compassion fatigue amongst colleagues have been documented.[54]

This lack of data back in 2019 was what initially motivated me to conduct the research central to this book. One aspect of the survey measured feelings of burnout among respondents. There are several tools for measuring burnout particularly in health care professionals, but I chose the Copenhagen Burnout Inventory which explores how people think how they have been feeling over the last two weeks.[55] It includes items on:

- Personal burnout (a state of prolonged physical and psychological exhaustion).

- Work related burnout (a state of prolonged physical and psychological exhaustion, which is perceived as related to the person's work).

- Client burnout (a state of prolonged physical and psychological exhaustion, which is perceived as related to the person's work with clients).

To score the questionnaire you consider how frequently participants experience these emotions. An average score of 50 or more relates to moderate burnout which equates to feeling all the symptoms sometimes (or of course some more often and some less as it is an average figure). An average score of 75 or more indicates high burnout, equating to experiencing those emotions most of the time.

For the personal burnout scale 60% of the survey respondents were considered to have moderate or above levels of personal burnout with 23% high levels. In terms of the proportion who felt these emotions or symptoms 'Always or often' over the last two weeks:

- Feeling tired: 74%
- Feeling physically exhausted: 52%
- Feeling emotionally exhausted: 87%
- Feeling that you can't take it anymore: 50%
- Feeling worn out: 87%
- Feeling weak and susceptible to illness: 54%

Although in part these symptoms could be explained by wider life factors such as chronic illness, caring responsibilities or home life challenges, the open-ended responses clearly showed that for some physical symptoms of exhaustion were role related:

> 'The last few years have taken their toll on my health and I feel very run down. I'm not as young as I was but I also think the role and political landscape is a lot harder these days.' (IBCLC)

> 'It differs from day to day but I feel I am increasingly having those days when I feel fraught and wrung out after yet more blocks and battles to simply do my job.' (Infant feeding lead)

For the work-related burnout scale 59% of survey respondents were considered to have moderate or above levels of personal burnout with 19% experiencing high levels. In terms of the proportion who felt these emotions or symptoms 'Always or often' over the last two weeks:

- Feeling that work is emotionally exhausting: 63%
- Feeling burnt out because of work: 40%
- Feeling frustrated by work: 56%
- Feeling worn out at the end of the working day: 91%
- Feeling exhausted in the morning at the thought of another day at work: 62%
- Feeling that every working hour is tiring: 50%
- Feeling enough energy for family and friends during leisure time: 52%

This frustration and exhaustion was evident across open ended responses:

> 'Some mornings I ask myself whether I can face another day of doing it all over again. I always do but I am angry about how it could easily not be this way if breastfeeding and supporting parents was properly respected.' (IBCLC)

> 'There seems to be too little time even to sleep properly or look after myself in other ways.' (Breastfeeding counsellor)

This presents a really concerning picture. Although you might expect those who are feeling more stressed and burned out to be more likely to complete a survey on mental health, skewing the data, these statistics are alarmingly high. Saying that, you might also conclude that those who are stressed may have less time to fill out such a survey, and those who are completely burned out may not feel motivated enough to take part meaning that these figures could even be underestimated. Whatever the explanation, the data are clear - a significant proportion of those working in lactation support are feeling burnt out in relation to their work tasks and feeling worn down and exhausted as a result of this.

However, there was a clear twist in the tale when it came to the core of the role for many – supporting families (I adapted the wording of the tool to use 'families' instead of the tool wording of 'clients'). Overall, only 8% were experiencing moderate to high levels of burnout here with just 1% showing high symptoms. For the specific items, the proportion of supporters who felt emotions 'Always or often' over the last two weeks was:

- Finding it hard to work with families: 5%
- Finding it frustrating to work with families: 5%
- Drained of energy by working with families: 9%
- Feeling that they give more than you they back when working with families: 5%
- Tired of working with families: 5%
- Wondering how long they will be able to continue working with families: 11%

There is a stark difference in the proportion of lactation supporters experiencing burnout symptoms in relation to supporting families compared to personal and work-related burnout, mirroring the earlier findings in relation to the emotional impact of the role. Stress and frustration are high but not with the 'actual' role or the motivation for entering the field in the first place. It is the bureaucracy, professional battles and lack of investment that surrounds it that leaves supporters so rundown.

It is also notable that the two items with the higher responses are personal i.e. feeling exhausted, rather than feeling tired of working with families. This was also clear in the open-ended responses. One breastfeeding counsellor eloquently described it as *'A rewarding job in a crappy environment.'* Others reflected on the juxtaposition between the reward and exhaustion of the role:

> *'The effects of my work sustain me emotionally. Even when I'm exhausted, spending time with a mother who suddenly feels a change in her breastfeeding boosts me for the next appointment.' (Breastfeeding counsellor)*

This pattern of findings is very similar to research in other caring professions. For example, in 2017 a survey exploring stress and burnout was sent to all members of the Royal College of Midwives in the UK. Almost 2000 midwives completed the survey with 83% reporting moderate and above levels of personal burnout and 67% moderate and above levels of work-related burnout.

However just 15% reported moderate levels of client-related burnout. Again, it was not the experience of working with families but broader system factors that were affecting midwives' wellbeing.[20] Likewise in an Australian study 57% of midwives were experiencing moderate to high levels of work and personal exhaustion but this fell to 9% for client-related burnout.[56]

As we saw earlier, symptoms of stress, anxiety and depression and burnout in similar professions such as midwifery are often higher amongst younger professionals.[56,57] In the survey data, levels of moderate to high burnout were also higher amongst those under 35, particularly those working as an IBCLC. Almost three quarters of younger IBCLCs had moderate to high levels of personal related burnout and two thirds were experiencing high levels of work related burnout.

Why? The higher likelihood of juggling small children with the role is possibly a key stressor but also the earlier years of any occupation can feel more stressful as you strive to find your place and client base. It has also been proposed that the shock of going from 'idealism' (where you truly hope you can save the breastfeeding world) to reality (where you realise there are many that you will not be able to change due to the system we are working in) can increase feelings of burnout.[20]

Conversely, many of those who were older in the survey had been in their role for decades. Logically, feelings of stress might be a little lower as a result of having adapted to and remained (survived?) in the role for all that time. However, it is possible that many of their peers who felt higher levels of stress left the profession and therefore did not take part.

Turning these statistics to personal stories it was clear that this stress was having an impact on the health and wellbeing of professionals and volunteers. Many respondents opened up about the physical and mental health complications they were experiencing:

'My job made me very ill - blood pressure 110 diastolic (I am fit active non-smoker non-drinker). I had anxiety, insomnia and a stomach ulcer. I took 3 months off sick and found another job but the difference was there were 2 of us in post not just me.' (Infant feeding lead)

'The stress sometimes makes me very ill. It is too much.' (Breastfeeding counsellor)

Although many in the survey were determined to continue to battle against the system because of their love of working with families, there were also poignant examples of once very motivated professionals who had reached the end of their tether and had nothing more left to give. Their responses were often brief and reflected the exhaustion and defeat that they felt. When examining their responses, what was stark was that these supporters also had high levels of client-related burnout. They no longer felt the protective buzz and satisfaction of working with families. Without that, the role lost all appeal.

'I am done and going through the motions. I'm counting down waiting for my moment to leave.' (Infant feeding lead)

'Achievements that once made me happy have no effect. In fact I struggle to even think of them as achievements. I feel very little in response to even the positive stories and know that means my days in what was once my vocation and passion are numbered. It is sad.' (Breastfeeding counsellor)

One participant in the survey explained how they had already stopped supporting breastfeeding. The survey was designed to explore the mental health of those working in lactation support, meaning it is likely that these voices are under-represented as those who had already left may not have taken part. It would be an important project to explore more of these voices in future research:

> 'I have lost my passion for breastfeeding and am taking a break because I hope it comes back in the future.' (Infant feeding advisor)

These cases of clear burnout are concerning and it's likely that many reading this book will see glimpses of themselves, even if just temporarily, in these words. Importantly however, they did not reflect the whole state of the profession. When asked about whether the stressors and pressures of working in lactation were impacting upon their ability to support women and continue in the role, only a relatively small proportion agreed. Overall, 10% felt that they 'were becoming numb to women's stories over time' and around 8% agreed that 'they often felt like giving it all up'. Clearly this is 8 - 10% too many. However, in contrast to the sheer number of participants who were battling stressors in the system, the desire to stay and fight is eye opening.

This leaves (at least) three important questions: why is this happening, why do we stay and what can we do about it? Over the next few chapters I will explore some of those challenges and stressors and reflect how the broader attitude to breastfeeding and perinatal health intertwines with this. Heads up – in some places it can be a tough (but also validating) read. If you're feeling overwhelmed, skip to the three later chapters which are a celebration of the work, the profession and you – 'Why we carry on', 'Tools for support' and 'A manifesto for change'.

Chapter 2

The impact of working in a system that doesn't value or support breastfeeding

'I do feel sometimes that I take the weight off a mother and carry it around myself. I worry about her long after she has left my care. I feel I carry the weights of all the women I have supported and the enormity of what we are fighting prevents me from putting them down.' (IBCLC)

It is clear from the previous chapter that many working and volunteering within the lactation field are struggling with feelings of burnout and stress, particularly in relation to the broader demands of the role. We know that this is reflective of how many working in healthcare professions feel, especially after Covid-19. All roles that involve the public, long hours and have an element of 'life or death' clearly have the potential to be stressful.

However, there are many additional factors about working in lactation support that add to the mix. Many are complex and difficult to unpick, and to some extent can be both challenging and motivating at the same time. Some, as we shall explore in more depth over the next few chapters, in part mirror the struggles that families face when wanting their baby to be breastfed. Essentially, you are trying to protect families from the pressures of the system, whilst also trying to navigate and fight that very same system yourself. Maybe this is a core element of why the work can elicit such feelings of frustration and overwhelm, but also empathy and compassion.

In the survey participants were asked about different aspects of their role that made their work challenging. It was clear that almost all participants were finding elements of the work distressing or overwhelming but predominantly that they were feeling worn down by aspects of their role that were often outside their control. It wasn't the core act of supporting breastfeeding and families that was so difficult, but rather a combination of the breastfeeding support landscape coupled with a tendency for a certain type of personality to gravitate towards this unique caring work. Indeed, returning to that reflection of the similarities between breastfeeding and being a breastfeeding supporter, often mothers will say *'It's not breastfeeding, I want a break from. It's balancing breastfeeding with everything else.'* Over the next few chapters, we will examine that 'everything else', hopefully providing additional validation as to why the role can feel so challenging (but also so worthwhile and necessary). In other words, it's not you - it's the system.

A lack of government investment in breastfeeding

'I fear until there is a health crisis that is directly linked back to lack of breastfeeding then the government isn't interested in investing in support. Unfortunately by then it will be too late.' (Peer supporter)

You would have to be hiding under a rock for the lack of investment and value in breastfeeding (and in new families in general) to pass you by. We know that many, if not most, of the challenges that women face when feeding their baby are due to factors at the system level that are outside their control. Despite government's supposedly promoting breastfeeding, that promotion is not often followed up by sufficient investment. A lack of resources for staffing, specialist roles and the infrastructure needed to provide high quality breastfeeding support leaves families struggling. Couple this with a multi-billion-dollar formula milk industry committed to undermining breastfeeding, and it's easy to see why so many stop breastfeeding before they are ready.[1]

In the survey just 7% of respondents felt that there had not been any cuts to breastfeeding support services in their local area in the last few years with half considering there to have been *'many cuts'* to what is offered. Some participants had been directly affected by these cuts with 10% having lost a paid position at some point, 14% a voluntary position and 18% both paid and voluntary work. As one peer supporter sadly noted *'I am being made redundant so our breastfeeding peer support service will end. No more training, no more groups, no more online support and no more volunteers'.*

Unfortunately, she was not alone. On top of that, over 94% were worried about future cuts to breastfeeding support posts and 96% were concerned over funding needed to deliver support such as a group venue. These worries are reinforced with 92% having witnessed more and more disinvestment in breastfeeding support services over time. Overall, 90% of survey respondents felt like they were fighting a *'losing battle against government cuts'.* This frustration was clear in open ended responses:

> *'I love breastfeeding support but have also got exhausted by the negative political landscape, which is a deliberate policy by this government. The biggest help would be respecting women's rights to breastfeed - which means proper leadership from the top, legislation to properly enact the WHO code, especially the avoidance of conflicted health professionals, plus funding for councils to rebuild community support.' (Breastfeeding counsellor)*

> *'It is demoralising when politicians sitting in their offices and who never see families reduce budgets or fail to support policy. They don't see the fall out in our communities yet hold all the power.' (IBCLC)*

Lactation professionals and supporters have to work within this system to try to do their best to pick up the pieces and fix the issues caused by a system that was meant to be protecting breastfeeding and families. This can make the role feel almost impossible at times. There are so many women and families to support, yet experts are often dismissed, underfunded and undervalued. Cuts to budgets and staffing seem to ever increase, whilst breastfeeding challenges increase, causing a feeling of battling against a failing system.

> *'We need more peer supporters, a clear pathway for women who need support, there is NO in-house support in the county I volunteer in... women travel over 1.5hrs for referrals on NHS.' (Peer supporter)*

> *'Families are driving over two hours in some cases to see me and I'm taking calls from all over. Sometimes I feel like I'm drowning as there is no one local to refer on to but plenty of providers I'd rather they avoid.' (IBCLC, Doula)*

Couple this lack of investment with a deep passion for breastfeeding and supporting families and an acute awareness of how damaging a difficult breastfeeding experience can be, and it's little wonder why so many in this field are feeling burnout and exhausted. A core part of this for many was feeling as if the work was not only never ending but ever increasing - three quarters of those in the survey believed that the situation and their role was becoming more and more challenging over time. Although some were able to find a semblance of work-life balance, for others this pressure was breaking them. The sheer number of families who needed support coupled with the passion and commitment of many working in the field is a dangerous game.

> *'I try to focus on those who I can help because if I allowed my brain to think about all those I cannot reach then I wouldn't get out of bed in the mornings.' (IBCLC)*

> *'There are too many families and too little of us. It is very stressful. The government needs to make more posts.' (Breastfeeding counsellor)*

In the survey participants were asked a series of questions around how their role in breastfeeding support fitted with family life and other commitments. The pattern of response was interesting in that overall, 89% of participants stated that they felt that their family understood the importance of breastfeeding support to them. However, although their family could see this passion and how vital it was, many also had concerns. Overall, 66% of respondents felt that their family thought they spent too much time giving breastfeeding support and 78% felt that their family thought that they worried too much about the state of breastfeeding, never able to fully switch off.

Participants also held these concerns themselves. Almost a third of respondents felt that they were not able to have clear cut family time where they did not offer any breastfeeding support and half of those with children found it hard to balance caring for them alongside the time they spent on breastfeeding support. Overall, two thirds worried that the time they spent on breastfeeding support took them away from family time and half agreed that they sometimes 'neglected' their partner if they had one as there is so much support they need to give elsewhere.

> *'I find it hard to switch off and not to give support when families need it. It has led to arguments with my partner as I've often one eye on my phone checking that everyone on the group is ok. I can see his point but I would feel terrible if I missed someone needing my help.' (Peer supporter)*

> *'I feel pressure from my husband that we are wasting what is supposed to be our retirement and we won't stay this fit forever.' (Peer supporter)*

For those who used social media as part of their breastfeeding role, it was clear that establishing boundaries was even more challenging. Almost half of participants struggled to regularly have 'rest days' where they didn't look at breastfeeding related social media, with fewer than a third of participants keeping to set hours when they gave support online. Over a third of participants also found that their online support got in the way of them being able to spend time relaxing.

When asked to estimate how many hours they were spending online (on social media or via messaging apps) giving support each week, although around half the sample estimated fewer than seven hours a week (equivalent to roughly an hour a day), others were clearly far more invested with around 10% of the sample spending on average more than three hours per day. Indeed, some participants were listing 40, 50 or even 60 hours per week with one participant estimating 12 hours per day, every day. This was often on top of providing face to face and phone/text support.

> 'It's hard to step away from helping people but the need is never ending. I think that I could spend my entire life, 24/7, responding to questions on social media and there would still be a huge backlog. I need to try and switch off and be stricter with myself because it's exhausting but I hate to think of parents out there worrying without a response. What if my delay meant someone stopped feeding?' (IBCLC)

> 'I'll spend the time in between appointments and groups answering chats and scrolling through groups posts. It's so easy to get carried away with how much support is given especially now we're all on our phones. It didn't used to be that way and I'm not sure whether that's a good or bad thing.' (IBCLC)

Many felt that they could not have a break from social media with over half of the respondents worried about the impact of this on personal and family boundaries. A quarter, predominantly those online every day for long periods, were worried that it was taking over their life. Additionally, more than half felt that their personal and professional identity had become blurred on social media. Online discussions often continued to play on people's minds long after they had closed their phone or laptop. Just a third of respondents felt that they were able to switch off mentally and forget about breastfeeding discussions they had online that day and less than a quarter were adept at ignoring social media notifications outside of working hours.

> *'I worry that I am addicted but it's hard to disconnect. The notifications keep coming at all hours.' (Peer supporter)*

> *'It would be easier to tell you when I'm not online to be honest. I'm not sure that's healthy though is it?' (Breastfeeding counsellor)*

The round the clock nature of the online world is a huge part of this issue. Whilst mothers often raise this as a benefit of online peer support,[2] for those doing the supporting it can be all consuming. There is also the issue of personal and professional lives becoming blurred with boundaries slowly dissolving.[3] Indeed, the sheer volume of time that could be spent online helping others has been raised in studies with other healthcare professionals.[4] Additionally, concerns around missing important information, seeing incorrect information posted online and fears about being perceived to be unprofessional are common amongst midwives who used social media.[5] Combined, these pressures lead us into spending more and more time online in a seemingly never ending anxiety overwork spiral.

Even with all this input and investment 87% of respondents found themselves *'often worrying about the mothers and babies that cannot be helped'*. Many could not stop thinking about parents outside of working hours or even long after they had left their care. On one hand this felt distressing and sometimes overwhelming. Supporters could not disentangle themselves from the emotional lives of others or escape to a place free from thoughts about breastfeeding. At the same time, this intensity and almost obsession with making things better was what drove supporters to continue. The complex irony of this was stark; in some ways it was the ineptitude of the system that both broke supporters whilst simultaneously fuelling their passion. The injustice of seeing women let down and babies not properly supported both exhausted them and gave them the fire to carry on.

This has been highlighted in research as a reason for many undertaking training in lactation in the first place – seeing so many families failed and so little investment in the system made women want to make a difference.[6] Remarkably, despite high levels of stress and burnout, when asked in the survey *'what is your first reaction when you hear about another cut to services or yet another breastfeeding mother having received poor advice'* almost two thirds of respondents stated that they still felt 'fired up and ready to try and change it'. Conversely, just 7% felt numb at such stories.

Clearly the profession is being run on the passion and determination of a group of motivated individuals. It is phenomenal to see, but is this not a risky strategy in the long term? Research into why individuals volunteer, or continue to work over their paid hours, shows that often it is because the role provides numerous personal rewards through feeling that you are making a difference, enjoying helping others and being part of a like-minded team. All true for many in the survey. However, a crucial element of feeling that reward is also feeling valued for the work you do. Caring and motivated people will go to the ends of the earth for something that is important to them but undervalue and disregard them and their positivity fades.[7] Is the reward from parents always going to be enough, even if the broader system continues to undervalue or criticise what many do?

Society does not value or understand breastfeeding

'We need a society that accepts the science about human milk, where we weren't having to go back to square one all the time in proving that it's important and deserves time and effort and resources. So much denial. Social media has made it worse because the misinformation spread is viral. Parents don't know what's real and what's not. Even medical providers are wading around in pseudoscience because it's what reinforces the reality they want to be true. Which is that it doesn't matter what you feed a baby. I had no idea how conflict laden this field would turn out to be and it exhausts me.' (IBCLC)

Sadly, it is not just governments who fail to see the importance of supporting breastfeeding. When asked in the survey whether they felt that the importance of breastfeeding was recognised, the response was overwhelmingly negative. Over 80% of participants in the survey agreed with statements that 'We are failing at convincing people that breastfeeding is important' and 'Many health professionals don't think breastfeeding is important'. On top of that, almost all participants felt that 'We are battling a society set up to fail breastfeeding women'. These statistics are pretty dismal and there's no getting away from that.

However, looking at it from a positive perspective, it was abundantly clear that once again for many respondents in the survey this was in fact this societal failing was what motivated them to get up and fight another day. As one IBCLC powerfully stated *'Society may not care for breastfeeding and breastfeeding mothers but I do – and I know my colleagues very much feel the same'*.

Trying to make a difference within this society that does not value or understand breastfeeding was a key source of frustration for those in the survey. Many participants talked about feeling like they were fighting a losing battle against a system of misperceptions and inaccurate information around feeding and caring for babies. It was exhausting to try to support a mother and give her good advice, only for a partner or friend or even an advert to convince her otherwise. Indeed, 96% of respondents in the survey felt frustrated at the amount of time they spent correcting misinformation. This was not just tedious but could be deeply upsetting. Almost all participants found it distressing to have to tell a mother that she had received incorrect information especially if it had damaged her breastfeeding journey. Many elaborated on this in the survey:

> *'There's only so much we can do. I try and do what I'm trained to do – give evidence-based information in a supportive and non-judgemental way. But sometimes it feels like everything works against me. I give support and then someone else gives a different message, often one that is easier to hear and we either end up unpicking all that or lose another mother to formula when that wasn't what she wanted.' (Peer supporter)*

Part of this frustration was the sheer 'Groundhog Day' nature of trying to fix the same issues over and over with 95% of participants feeling that it felt like they encountered the same issues daily. This repetition of fixable issues was described as demoralising, especially when attempts had been made to correct information or unhelpful ways of practice in a local area and yet the same misinformation or poor care kept repeating itself.

> *'I am so fed up of seeing the same issues over and over when we know how to fix them.' (IBCLC)*

> *'I can predict what challenges women at our group will be facing and that's not because I'm a magical fortune teller but because breastfeeding support is depressingly predictable.' (Peer supporter)*

Another inevitable aspect of trying to work in a society that doesn't understand or value breastfeeding is the continual feeling of pressure to create a safe haven away from all the misinformation and criticism that new parents face. Many professionals and volunteers were working with women and families who were making a different choice by breastfeeding than their family and friends did. Although some parents had support in theory from family and friends in their decision to breastfeed, many still faced challenges from being given incorrect information such as 'if you move to formula he'll sleep better' or being ridiculed, reflecting broader research on this issue.[8]

The support that these families needed to breastfeed became more than simple information and encouragement – they desperately needed validation and reassurance that they were not strange, unusual, or being selfish in their feeding choice. This reflects previous research which highlighted how mothers feel that breastfeeding peer support groups can feel like a safe space away from criticism[1] and that this 'safe space' is something that IBCLCs strive to achieve for those they are caring for.[9]

'I've been told several times that I'm a lifesaver or lifeline for mothers and it shouldn't be this way. What I'm doing isn't rocket science in a lot of cases and it can feel like I'm being paid to give what feels like simple information to me. What I am doing I guess is being their constant and a trusted source of information and it is that which is invaluable to them amongst all the noise and criticism.' (IBCLC)

'I feel an intense need to protect mothers and create that place where they can feel they belong.' (Peer supporter)

On a more personal level this lack of understanding of the breastfeeding and lactation role often led to confusion during *'and what is it you do?'* work-related conversations. Friends and family reacted in a variety of ways, considering the role to be unusual, bizarre or even made up. More on this later when we reflect on the 'loneliness of the lactation professional' but this reaction left respondents feeling underappreciated and even mocked by those close to them. Meanwhile volunteers often felt as if people thought their work was not important or a 'real' role because it was not paid, despite the hard work and long hours that went into supporting families.

'I'm not even entirely sure that my husband fully appreciates what my job entails and certainly extended family meet ups can be awkward when an unsuspecting distant relative asks me how work is going.' (IBCLC)

'My husband once called it my hobby. He was swiftly put straight but that stung. Oh how I wish it was a carefree pastime.' (Peer supporter)

Female health care is underfunded and undervalued

You'd think the fact that everybody was once a baby and many will go on to care for babies would mean that breastfeeding would be seen as an important issue across the health spectrum. Couple this with the research studies that show how much unsupported infant feeding decisions can ultimately cost health systems, it should be a subject of great public interest. Right? Well of course we know it's sadly not. Despite its relevance, the importance of breastfeeding is often missing from many policies and government round table discussions and is usually far from being a topic deemed worthy of social conversation.

Indeed, when we look back at the history of how breastfeeding support emerged as a 'role' in the first place, it was due to women essentially deciding that they had had enough of society working against breastfeeding, or governments refusing to invest in it. Women have always supported other women to breastfeed, but more 'formalised' groups grew from them taking matters into their own hands by setting up mother to mother support groups or networks in communities. For example, the story behind the formation of La Leche League describes how two women - Mary White and Marian Tompson -

were so fed up with poor support for breastfeeding mothers that they got together a group of friends to understand more about breastfeeding and support other women. The international organisation grew from there.[10]

Other support groups and initiatives have also grown from within communities to specifically meet the needs of the women, parents and families within them. Globally, numerous different groups occur in different formalities, many with a focus on reaching those in more marginalised or underserved groups, or those who were not represented in some of the first more formalised groups such as those living in deprived communities, Indigenous women, Women of Colour and with LGBTQ identities.

Whilst community led initiatives are undoubtedly feminist and empowering, they also shine a light on the problematic issue that healthcare should not be left to volunteers. Although there is funding available and it is possible to make lactation support a career, support is heavily propped up by the goodwill of volunteers (as we shall explore in more depth later). Infant feeding is relevant to us all, yet as our day-to-day realities and the survey data show us, so often it relies on a small number of highly motivated individuals, *predominantly* women, giving up their time and expertise, often having their own other work and caring responsibilities to juggle.

We know that when we attend conferences, the majority of attendees are female. When we do get the support of politicians and policy makers, the majority are female. What is it about this subject that a) relies on the good will of women and b) seemingly disinterests or scares away most men? Anger at this was reflected strongly. It was felt that support for infant feeding was left to women to sort out, and often volunteers at that.

'Relying on female volunteers isn't fair and the government needs to own health promotion by financing it.' (IBCLC, HCP)

> *'IBCLCs are worth their weight but are practically invisible both inside and outside the NHS. All women should have an IBCLC assigned to her care to walk alongside her for at least the first six weeks of her baby's life. Someone specialist in identifying lactation challenges with time to dedicate to supporting each and every woman and baby, could transform our miserable breastfeeding rates. I don't think it would be that expensive either - not compared to what the NHS spends on treating illness both short and long which are a result of not breastfeeding. Economically it's a no brainer. My cynicism says it's because it's a woman's issue that there's so little investment - invisible, with no voice and not enough influence.' (IBCLC)*

Sadly, we know that female healthcare, particularly around reproduction and sexual health receives a tiny proportion of the funding that male healthcare receives - with research into transgender and non-binary reproductive health practically non-existent. Five times more research is conducted into erectile dysfunction – a condition that affects 19% of men – compared with premenstrual syndrome, which affects 90% of women.[11] Meanwhile the Better Births Maternity Services Review in the UK highlighted how perinatal health research is still majorly underfunded.[12]

This is exacerbated when it comes to perinatal health, particularly breastfeeding, as there is little direct 'profit' for investors to make. When you think of investments into breastfeeding they are often around products and the big money isn't for everyday products either. Large sums have been invested into nipple shields that measure milk intake[13] and even trying to replicate components of breast milk in lab produced milk.[14] Breastfeeding support? Not so much. Meanwhile the global breast milk substitute industry is now worth over 55 billion USD.[15]

> *'It's depressing to realise how much more formula companies have to play with.' (IBCLC)*

This underinvestment culture makes both breastfeeding and supporting breastfeeding even more difficult. In her talk *'Approaching care when you're barely there: Re-imagining empathy when you've got nothing left to give'* Nekisha Killings MPH, IBCLC talks about the challenge of supporting breastfeeding and showing empathy to families within a patriarchal culture that adopts male centric perspectives on health, care and empathy.[16]

A male healthcare dominated system tends to focus on illnesses that affect middle aged men, research data that adopts the medical model such as that from well-funded randomised controlled trials, and solutions that are based around clinical intervention, medication and profit.[17] This is not exactly what lactation support, relational care and women and family centred approaches are all about, to say the least! There's no immediate profit, or money-making product, from successfully supporting breastfeeding – and this is reflected in the lack of investment. Meanwhile, governments appear blind to the long-term cost savings from investing in perinatal health and infant feeding in particular.

In survey responses, this challenge was also felt to be exacerbated by the lactation profession being a predominantly female-led career. Although men do work within the field, their numbers are relatively low (with just one male respondent in the survey). Although there are of course exceptions, occupations that are predominantly female led have lower rates of pay and prestige compared to their equivalent male role.[18]

'If this issue was affecting men in the same way we'd have breastfeeding support on tap. I think the government fully understands that we are crying out for help but doesn't care because it's women who are affected.' (Peer supporter)

The reliance on volunteers to support infant feeding also ties in with the wider issue of women, unpaid labour and caring roles. We know that despite an increase in women's participation in the workplace since the 1980s, women still take on the majority of unpaid labour and caregiving at home and in the community and this has increased hugely during the Covid-19 pandemic.[19] Dubbed 'the second shift' by Hochschild back in 1989, many women juggle a full or part time role combined with more than half the housework and caring responsibilities back home.[20]

Although of course there are many variations in how couples split responsibilities, overall women are more likely to experience something called 'family-work spillover' or in other words school are more likely to call them when their child falls over in the playground despite their male partner being listed as first contact. This 'disruption' is so common that it is considered normal.[21]

This can be particularly challenging in caring professions. Your work demands that you are emotionally present and many of the families that you work with will have complex emotional stories. This can be rewarding but also draining work, especially when women also end up taking on a greater share of the emotional needs of their family, including the unseen emotional load. In one study of nurses with young families many talked about needing to be continually 'attentive' to competing needs (i.e. what do I desperately need to do for my work today but also when am I going to create that costume for my child's octopus themed dress up day that school have announced with three days notice). Flexibility was also mentioned a lot.[22] Or in plain English terms – how do I do all the things at once without dropping too many balls, at least not the ones that really matter?

Take home message: Working in lactation support can feel like an uphill battle because it is. You are fighting against a system that often undervalues breastfeeding, mothers and new families. Fires have to be put out and problems fixed before you can start at the beginning. In other words, it's not you - it's the system (but please carry on fighting it, we will overthrow it eventually).

Chapter 3

Passion, empathy and our own challenging feeding experiences

'Seeing a mother have to stop breastfeeding is like a knife through my heart.' (Peer supporter)

Lactation support is a strange place to work sometimes (hah! *'Only sometimes?!'* I hear you say). You work within a system that often doesn't understand the importance of what you do. It's underfunded and under-resourced. Friends, family and society sometimes don't get why you do what you do, or simply don't understand what it is you do at all. It can be a very lonely place, and one that seems to attract more than its fair share of conflict (more on these points later in the book). So why on earth do so many of us just keep on keeping on? In short, because of our passion to protect the families we work with and support.

…Scrabbling around for money to run a group? No problem, we'll work around it.

…Yet another article printed in a newspaper decrying the importance of breastfeeding? No problem, it'll be tomorrow's fish and chip paper.

…A colleague who questions your entire existence? Meh, no problem, who cares what they think anyway?

All of that is just noise in a vocation that people are deeply drawn to, often because of their own past experiences and who they are. The wider role may be deeply frustrating, but we know why we do it and who we do it for. It's almost visceral and something we can't always directly put into words. At the same time, it is this passion and commitment that in part makes our lives so challenging. I will take a guess and say for many reading this book, the work can feel so tough because of how much you care.

…You care about women, parents, babies and families
…You care about breastfeeding
…You care about society and our future
…You care about correct information and evidence
…You care about your colleagues and doing a good job
…You care about making a difference

Combined with the injustice that is the lack of investment in perinatal health alongside our own infant feeding experiences, some days it just all feels too much. Ironically, it is the fact that you care so much that makes you so good at what you do. I'll visit strategies for coping with the stress of the role later, but for now, read on and see if you recognise yourself in any of the following.

Human milk: Human kindness

'I feel hurt when mothers are hurt by bad information.'
(Breastfeeding counsellor)

Empathy is the ability to recognise, feel and even experience the emotions of others. It has three elements. You can experience affective empathy (the ability to respond to other people's emotions appropriately), somatic empathy (the ability to feel what another person is feeling) and cognitive empathy (the ability to understand someone's emotional reaction). People with high levels of empathy tend to have the following traits:

- A desire to help other people
- A tendency to think a lot about how other people feel
- A good ability to recognise how others are feeling
- A radar for spotting lies
- Caring deeply for those around them
- Excellent listening skills

Empathy is an important tool for those working in occupations that support others and is particularly high amongst health care professionals. Nurses and midwives show some of the strongest levels of empathy, with female professionals having the highest overall scores.[1] Empathy is integral to the compassionate care that centres families. In has been linked to improved birth satisfaction[2] and supporting parents through difficult situations such as baby loss.[3] Meanwhile, we know that empathetic listening and support during the postnatal period can help reduce symptoms of postnatal depression and birth trauma.[4]

Research has also highlighted the importance of receiving emotional support from health professionals and supporters for continued breastfeeding.[5] Mothers value personal care that is sensitive to their individual needs.[6] Interventions that focus on supporting mothers holistically and exploring their wider context are more likely to result in mothers feeling supported.[7] Peer supporters in particular are valued for the care, connection and empathy that they provide to new mothers.[8] So all good, right?

Kind of. Like many psychological phenomena, some empathetic ability is a good thing, but experiencing too little or too much can be detrimental. Empathy is a social tool. It allows us to connect to others and develop supportive relationships. However, if you have too much empathy you absorb the weight of other people's problems which is exhausting. Although those skills listed above are great for working in a supportive role, it often has a personal cost. People high in empathy tend to:

- Feel drained by too much social connection
- Feel overwhelmed around a lot of people
- Feel distressed by the suffering of others
- Find it difficult to set boundaries

As you might imagine empathy is a double-edged sword in lactation support. Often, it's precisely why people end up in this field in the first place. You recognise just how much support others need and how important it is to them because you can understand and feel their emotions. You're skilled at responding in the way that they need. The families that you work with value that and keep coming back. You're their safe place. The one that understands how they feel in a society that disregards and demeans what they are doing. And that feels amazing. SO amazing. Indeed, the euphoria a good day can bring was illustrated throughout survey responses:

'I love, love, love helping a mother get it right.' (Peer supporter)

'There is no better feeling than seeing a happy, smiling mother walk out your door.' (IBCLC)

However, because of the pressures in infant feeding support, giving all that support and responding to the stories and needs of parents can be emotionally exhausting. You absorb the stress and heartbreak they are feeling and because so many parents are let down, there's a lot to take in. This in turn starts to affect your wellbeing. Indeed, in the survey 85% of respondents said that they felt *'Guilty if a mother they were caring for cannot be supported to continue breastfeeding'* and 82% felt significant *'Distress at telling a woman that she might need to stop breastfeeding'*.

'The worst part for me is when women stop and are distraught by that. Even if it's nothing I have done I feel responsible and it's an awful feeling.' (IBCLC)

'My heart has broken alongside so many mothers over the years.' (Breastfeeding counsellor)

It will come as little surprise that high levels of empathy are linked to higher levels of compassion fatigue, burnout and general exhaustion.[9] It's a seemingly never-ending circle of caring so much that you want to support parents, but the outcome of seeing all those stories and giving all that support means that you inevitably end up caring even more. It can feel like there's no escape, which is probably why so many of the respondents in the survey said that they felt they could never take a proper break. Throw in the fact that high levels of empathy put you at higher risk of vicarious trauma[10] (trauma from watching traumatic events continually happen to others - we'll return to this later) and it's no surprise so many are struggling.

Stats nerd interlude coming up here for a moment on the complicated relationship between empathy and burnout data. If you read some studies they suggest that lower levels of empathy are linked to a higher rate of burnout. This is a good example of the difference between two things being linked to each other (i.e. correlation) and considering whether one caused the other or not (i.e. causation). Some studies just take a snapshot of experience. Usually however when low empathy is linked to burnout, what is in fact going on is that over time burnout can have the effect of reducing empathy levels.[11] It's not that high empathy levels protect against burnout, but rather burnout can wear down ability to empathise.[12]

If the researchers in those types of paper had conducted a longitudinal study, then they may likely have seen the pattern of high empathy levels at the start, falling over time as symptoms of burnout rose. Essentially this high level of empathy for others can make us prone to giving too much of ourselves to the role as we feel so deeply for families involved. However, that sustained investment often unfortunately ends with us feeling exhausted and burnt out.[13]

There have been numerous studies looking at empathy rates in other healthcare professionals[14] with one study recognising (but not measuring) a high level of empathy amongst IBCLCs.[15] But what did empathy levels look like in this data? As part of the survey participants completed a measure that looks at the ability to recognise and understand emotions in others.[16] It has a potential score from 20 – 100 with the average score of the population typically being around 50.[17] Those working in health care and caring positions do tend to have a higher level of empathy than the general population. In the survey data the score of the 'least' empathetic participant was 55, with an average score of 79. A third of the sample scored above 80 reflecting a very high level of empathy.

Basically, everyone who took part had a higher level of empathy than average, with many topping the scale. It turns out we certainly do care, which let's face it is not actually a revelation but it's nice to see it in real figures. But do we care too much for our own sakes? Or is being highly empathetic something we actually enjoy and a vital part of what makes us so suited to the breastfeeding support role? I think only you can decide what your own personal boundaries are, but I do know that making time to also care for yourself even half as much as you care for others is important. We'll revisit this in the later chapter about supporting your wellbeing.

The role of our own challenging feeding experiences

'I have a need to ensure that no other person goes through what I went through. Nobody should have to, and I can help prevent that.' (IBCLC)

A common criticism seen on social media or in the press is that those working in the lactation field are often fanatics, determined to promote only breastfeeding at the expense of everything else. It's often assumed (by people who have no idea what they are talking about) that everyone working in breastfeeding support had a lovely, easy experience and simply doesn't understand the struggles that other people face. That's why we want them to breastfeed – to be just like us! To skip through the fields of daisies happily nursing our babies. Sheer bliss! Right…?

Often this could not be further from the truth. Many working in lactation support are there precisely because they have struggled and had difficult experiences.[18] They may also have really struggled to find support. They may have needed to introduce formula or stop before they were ready. They carry the pain and grief of those experiences around with them and it's because of these experiences that they want to help others.[19] Others may have had positive experiences and know the difference someone knowledgeable and supportive can make to an infant feeding journey. Out of all the responses in the survey this need to protect others and to try to ensure that they didn't experience the same trauma was one of the most common themes:

> *'Seeing mothers struggling breastfeeding their baby and the hard work that they put in, makes me feel that I would like to help them, as I went through the hardship and I don't want another mother having the same hardship.'* (Breastfeeding counsellor)

As professionals and supporters, we know how traumatising a difficult or prematurely ended breastfeeding experience can be. Knowing that breastfeeding difficulties and stopping before you are ready can increase risk of postnatal depression,[20] feelings of failure and guilt,[21] and long-lasting feelings of grief[19] is what motivates us and keeps us awake at night. Simultaneously we know what a positive breastfeeding experience can mean in terms of maternal wellbeing, identity and mothering experience.[22] And we don't just know this – we care about making a difference to that. This played out in the survey data with 93% of respondents agreeing that they were *'Worried about mothers' wellbeing in an underfunded system'*.

This deeply caring nature is reflected in research examining mothers' perceptions of breastfeeding peer supporters. One qualitative study with new mothers into the breastfeeding care they had received found that they described peer supporters as 'caring', 'enthusiastic' and 'encouraging'.[23] This recognition is often important to peer supporters who take deep pride and value in perceiving that mothers genuinely felt that supporters really cared about them and their breastfeeding experience.[24] In another qualitative study exploring the perceptions of women, health professionals and peer supporters of the peer supporter role, the level of empowerment, hope and reassurance offered by peer supporters was clear. Many acted as peers and friends supporting families across all aspects of parenting and not just breastfeeding.[25]

Indeed, a major part particularly of the peer supporter role is providing emotional support and connection with mothers and families. Research (and our own personal stories) show us that women value how caring and empathetic peer supporters can be, knowing that they understand and have experienced what the mother is going through. Women value hearing peer supporters' own experiences of breastfeeding including the difficulties they experienced and overcame. Peer supporters are viewed as honest and are 'telling you what it's really like' which helps women connect and bond with supporters.[26]

This relational approach to breastfeeding support is also visible throughout the care of lactation consultants, although there is relatively little research documenting this work compared to other professions. In her PhD thesis, entitled *'Managing connection and disconnection: relationship as the centre of Lactation Consultant care for breastfeeding women and their babies'*, Dr Jennifer Hocking explored the central focus of relationships within the IBCLC role. Empathy, kindness and gentleness were integral to the role with an emphasis on creating supportive and nurturing environments often within busy practice spaces.[15] Likewise, in another interview study with IBCLCs the importance of being woman centred and addressing a mother's emotional needs and broader experience of caring for her baby alongside any practical breastfeeding guidance was felt to be central to the role.[27]

This emotion work, no matter how satisfying and rewarding, is however recognised as tiring and labour intensive. It is not something that you can walk away from easily, not least when you meet mothers who are living an experience that reflects your own. When they struggle or stop breastfeeding before they are ready and feel all the emotions that can bring, you can feel them too, in addition to a deep need and feeling of responsibility to support them. The weight of these stories over time can feel heavy, especially for those whose circumstances you may feel powerless to fix.

> *'Sometimes a mother's story makes me catch my breath because it is word for word my own. It physically hurts me to hear.' (IBCLC)*

> *'I can feel frantic when I know I cannot help a mother. It's an awful feeling.' (Breastfeeding counsellor)*

The depth and breadth of breastfeeding grief can lead to vicarious trauma

Vicarious trauma (known also as secondary trauma) can occur when health and social care professionals witness distressing events happening to the patients and clients that they are caring for. As with post-traumatic stress disorder it can have a catastrophic impact upon wellbeing including feelings of despair, grief and depression.[28] Vicarious trauma is closely linked to compassion fatigue and burnout from the toll of frequently seeing those that you are supporting experiencing negative events or poor care despite your best intentions.[29]

Research is growing in understanding the related field of how birth trauma can impact upon those caring for women.[30] For example, research has explored the concept of midwives as 'second victims' to a traumatic birth.[31] Midwives who have witnessed traumatic births, often repeatedly, can be left with feelings of self-blame, guilt and self-doubt even if they had done everything that they could to alleviate the situation.[32]

Over time vicarious trauma can affect personal relationships, impact negatively upon mental health and cause midwives to want to leave the profession.[33] Midwives can feel so connected to the trauma of the women they were caring for that it is as if they went through the event themselves.[34] It is not uncommon for healthcare professionals who have experienced birth related vicarious trauma to experience flashbacks and other intrusive memories of events.[30]

Although research has not yet explored vicarious trauma as a concept specifically in relation to breastfeeding support roles, it is clear that it is occurring. One research study with midwives highlighted the guilt that many can feel when they want to support breastfeeding but simply do not have the time or staffing levels to be able to do so properly. When women in their care then struggle and experience difficulties or stop breastfeeding before they are ready, midwives recount how the experience is 'heart-breaking', 'soul-destroying' and 'distressing'.[35] This was clearly seen in responses:

> 'I would go as far as to say I have been left traumatised by the stories of some women. It takes a long time to process and work through and I'm not sure I truly forgive myself even if I did everything I could.' (IBCLC)

As previously discussed, one of the frustrations that many lactation supporters carry is the experience of being dismissed by other healthcare professionals, or their guidance being ignored or overruled. These experiences, when coupled with distressing outcomes, have been linked to an increased risk of vicarious trauma. In research with midwives, anger and distress were common responses to having to follow guidance that they did not agree with, or ideas or advice being overridden.[36]

Likewise, student midwives who were observers at traumatic births and unable to step in felt significant guilt, despite not being responsible for the situation.[37] Others were negatively affected by feeling helpless when they couldn't help with issues such as domestic violence.[38] In the survey the experience of picking up the pieces after a woman had received inaccurate information was all too common and frustrating. Others talked about how they spent time with women carefully preparing feeding plans and supporting them, only to come back in the morning and find everything had been overridden by staff on a night shift or by a medical professional.

'I'm fed up of my careful support and instructions being overridden when I go off shift or someone senior comes in and goes against everything I have said, even though I know my guidance was evidence based and correct.' (Midwife)

'The consistency with which GPs around here repeatedly give poor information to mothers which ends with them giving up feeding is shocking. No matter how much I reassure them that they do not need to stop to take a certain medication it's ignored because they assume that the GP knows best.' (Health visitor)

Take home message: This role can feel tough because you care so much. It is important and it matters to you because often you know how much difference the right lactation support can mean. This deep empathy and ability to connect makes you who you are, but it can also eat away at you as you have a tendency to put others before yourself. Remember to treat yourself as you treat those you care for - with kindness and compassion and give yourself permission to take a break!

Chapter 4

The stress of disconnection and conflict

'Thank you for asking about our wellbeing. It's nice to know that someone cares. I quite often feel that most people don't.' *(Peer supporter)*

Who you work alongside can make all the difference to a job. Even the most mundane and soulless positions can be made enjoyable by feeling part of a team and connected to others, whereas our dream positions can become hellish due to 'challenging' working relationships. Earlier in the book I touched briefly on the concepts of isolation and loneliness in terms of feeling misunderstood and undervalued by peers and wider society when it comes to supporting lactation. As with other parts of the survey findings, the sections exploring relationships and support within lactation presented a very mixed pattern, with many respondents feeling both connected and disconnected to others in their world.

Positively, many respondents felt that they had at least one person that they could turn to for support and that made a huge difference to their resilience and determination to carry on, with fewer than 10% of respondents feeling totally isolated. This individual often acted as a lifeline, shielding against the stress and negativity that others and the role could bring. For example, 85% of participants agreed that they had *'at least one good friendship in lactation support to offload to'* and two thirds felt *'part of a larger community of peers, with whom I can openly share my concerns and questions'.*

> *'When I'm with others who understand it's like an injection of energy.' (Infant feeding lead)*

> *'The support I have from my colleagues (LLL leaders) keeps me going.' (Breastfeeding counsellor)*

I return to the important and protective nature of these connections in more depth in chapter seven 'Why we carry on'. However, it was also clear that alongside these positive relationships, broader interactions were more mixed. There was often a significant split between feeling connected and valued by those working in roles that understood infant feeding but a large disconnect with those who did not. Regarding the latter, many respondents felt unsupported, criticised or undervalued by some colleagues or troubled by broader online criticisms and fall out and bullying between peers. Let's look at which aspects were specifically difficult and why.

The role can be lonely

Although many in the survey felt a strong connection with other infant feeding specialists and their peers, when thinking about their broader health professional colleagues over a third felt '*very alone professionally*'. This was typical amongst those who were the infant feeding lead within their team when others did not fully support or prioritise breastfeeding.

> '*Sometimes in larger teams I feel very lonely and misunderstood by other professionals who do not understand the importance and relevance of infant feeding across early development.*' (Infant feeding lead)

> '*I feel powerless and left to my own devices. I work in a team however I am very much not part of the "team". I'm a lone worker and have a different role and that is very much known. I'm looked down upon and treated very differently. It can be so lonely some days and so difficult when sometimes all you are doing is fixing problems.*' (Maternity support worker)

This was also true for some working in private practice. Although many felt connected to a broader community of peers, some rarely saw anyone else in day-to-day life except of course those families they were supporting. There was no shared office or workplace to attend or colleagues to work alongside or have a tea break with. Although some enjoyed this independence and more introverted working approach, others missed the collegiality and company of others.

> *'I left a hospital based team to work for myself and I mostly enjoy it but sometimes I can go for weeks without seeing anyone else on a professional level.' (IBCLC)*

> *'When something goes wrong I particularly miss having the support of a team. It can feel that you are very alone and that is distressing.' (IBCLC)*

Professional conflict can be common

Alongside feeling different or isolated, some respondents experienced conflict and anxiety in their relationships with colleagues and other professionals that they worked alongside. This made the job feel so much tougher than it needed to be and contributed to feelings of loneliness and a lack of support. A quarter of respondents felt strongly that the wider health system that they were working in did not understand their role or its value, and over half felt undermined in their role by other colleagues. Fewer than half of respondents felt that other health professionals working in their local area valued them, although this was context dependent. While a lactation consultant, for example, often felt valued and supported in lactation settings, in other multidisciplinary teams they felt some professions looked down on them.

> *'I cannot get one local GP to accept my training and experience. He keeps dismissing information that I provide to mothers and the surgery as if I have no idea what I am talking about.' (IBCLC)*

> *'Women love and appreciate my support, but my colleagues and management consistently undermine the value of infant feeding. If I support women, I'm seen as going rogue... this is exhausting.' (IBCLC)*

A core part of this conflict was often being perceived as unusual, strange or even 'nasty' because of a passion for supporting breastfeeding and families. Many felt unfairly denigrated simply for this, with some commenting that it was surreal to be disliked simply for wanting a better future for families. Others were simply dismissed or treated with an almost kindly 'othering', whilst some felt this effect far more sharply with disparaging or nasty comments being made about their work.

> *'It is lonely work and that feels upsetting. How can anyone dislike someone who dedicates their life to making things better?' (IBCLC)*

> *'I have been criticised and it suggested that I am shaming parents by others in the health board. It is unfair and uncalled for and most of all not true.' (Peer supporter)*

This was heightened and often acrimonious in nature if there had been conflict in the past over information given to parents. This difficult working relationship often arose as a consequence of parents being given outdated, or non-evidence-based information about infant feeding, or wider parenting issues such as sleep routines. Lactation supporters felt that they had to step in to support the parents with accurate information often at the expense of their relationship with a colleague or other professional. This often led to conflict or a cooling of working relationships. As a result, three quarters of survey respondents found it stressful to have to 'correct' or intervene when they saw other healthcare professionals give poor information.

'I'm sick to the back teeth of having to be the bad guy who intervenes and corrects senior staff who consistently give out bad info. It causes bad vibes and is somehow my fault even though they are the ones in the wrong.' (IBCLC)

'I got a lot of stick for questioning the information a GP and me referring the mother instead to Breastfeeding Network information but ultimately I was right and at the end of the day the mother I was supporting could carry on breastfeeding and I'm not sorry for that.' (Peer supporter)

On the theme of acceptance, another common experience was the tension between lactation consultants who were also qualified healthcare professionals and those who had entered the field through different pathways. Those without a nursing or other healthcare background often felt 'second best' or not considered to be real professionals allowed to work within hospital settings.

'I've considerable experience of supporting probably thousands of families over the years but I will never be able to get a hospital based role as I do not have a nursing qualification. I don't want to provide nursing care, I want to provide lactation expertise and am as good as, or even better than those who can be employed in those roles. How is this two-tier system fair? It's divisive and prevents me from helping families.' (IBCLC)

This issue is of course complex, and we will return to it in chapter nine when considering the manifesto for change. A balance needs to be found between maximising opportunity for lactation professionals to work across settings whilst also ensuring that other aspects of clinical care are upheld. Not every lactation role within a health service requires broader healthcare training but some roles will. As always, I think the answer here would be to 'build a bigger table' and have more posts with varied applicants and backgrounds. Wouldn't that be nice!

Peer supporters often had a very varied experience working alongside others in the team, depending very much on who they were working with. On the one hand, many shared positive stories of acceptance and collaborative working, feeling that they fitted in well with other professionals and were valued:

'I'm really lucky in my area as I feel really valued by the health visitor who leads our group. She's fab and makes us feel like we're really part of the team.' (Peer supporter)

'I was asked by a midwife to train in this role and I have to say it made me really proud and a bit excited to get to work alongside her and the rest of the team.' (Peer supporter)

'I know the local team have my back and that's a big part of why I feel confident in what I do to support families.' (Peer supporter)

However, others were brought down by being dismissed or undervalued by some in the team, with three quarters feeling undermined by (a minority of) other health professionals in their role.

'I've gained so much knowledge over the years but many of the health professionals treat me like I'm still just another mum. I know they value some parts of what I do but I do also know what I'm talking about around basic breastfeeding care. I'm not saying I should run the group instead of them but please allow me to share what I have learned with others and not jump in when I'm asked a question I easily know the answer to.' (Peer supporter)

'I know what I'm talking about but I work with some people who think only they can help with breastfeeding and I should be confined to giving tea, saying "there, there" and referring back to them. Despite having been a peer supporter for 10 years with huge amounts of success.' (Peer supporter)

Research exploring the relationships between peer supporters and other health care professionals can unfortunately reveal mixed findings. Taking the positives first - research has identified how rewarding, supportive and successful collaborative working can be. Peer supporters can lighten the load and both peer supporters and healthcare professionals can learn valuable experiences from each other.[1] When relationships are mutually respectful and roles understood there is real value in collaborative working.[2] Others have found that although it can take a while for a relation to develop, once established both groups find collaboration beneficial.[3]

However, just like with most other working relationships there is the risk of conflict. Some research has found that sometimes peer supporters feel undermined or that their skills are dismissed because they are not in healthcare roles. In one qualitative study exploring experiences of breastfeeding peer supporters, some felt that health professionals did not fully understand their role. Others felt undermined and not accepted by health care professionals, leaving them feeling like 'outsiders'. Others felt that there was a clear divide between the 'real' professionals and peer supporters that caused a hierarchy of role and experience when in fact skills were often complementary.[4] This is an important conversation to take further. Although clearly many organisations deeply value their peer supporters, what training and communication is needed to support some to recognise how experiences and skills complement each other so that all can thrive?

Impostor syndrome is exacerbated by conflict

'You've got to try to believe in yourself as there are plenty who will not.' (Peer supporter)

A continual feeling of being criticised or undermined can lead to impostor syndrome developing even in the most confident individual. Impostor syndrome is the feeling that you don't belong or deserve to be in your role and emerges from the belief that you simply don't have enough knowledge, skill, or experience to be doing what you're doing. Sometimes it stops us from taking opportunities in the first place and other times it gives us that continual looking over our shoulder, waiting to be caught out feeling when we're in a role or creating something. It has been described as 'waiting for the tap on the shoulder' – for someone who is a 'real expert' (or 'grown up'?) to come and break the news that everyone has realised that you're nowhere near qualified for the role and would you please now leave.

If you're experiencing impostor syndrome you might believe that your work is just not a good enough standard, or that everyone knows better than you. You might struggle with offering information, suggesting new ideas or leading on new initiatives. You may think that you'll never be good enough or feel that everything you do must be perfect. This can be particularly tricky in a field like lactation support as you know that the stakes are high. You might be feeling the weight of knowing that the support you are able to give a family might make or break breastfeeding for them, or doubting your training and expertise. It can also feel like there is a long queue waiting to tell you that you're doing it wrong or shouldn't even exist in the first place.

Impostor syndrome is common amongst health care professionals. One study found that around a third of health care students scored highly on imposter syndrome symptoms.[5] However, when studies take into account sex, this rises sharply for women with research suggesting that almost half of female healthcare students experience impostor syndrome.[6] Unfortunately this doesn't go away with time and experience. Data shows that impostor syndrome can persist through qualification all the way through to senior health care staff.[7]

Impostor syndrome isn't a nice thing to experience in itself and is associated with an increased risk of anxiety, depression, low self-esteem and burnout.[8] It is also linked to a less favourable work-life balance. People with stronger feelings of impostor syndrome are more likely to feel that they need to work all hours, either to do enough or to prove their worth. Many feel as if they have to be better than everyone else, and work harder simply to be considered 'good enough'.[9]

So how did those in the survey feel? Participants were asked a series of questions around the concept of impostor syndrome. Overall, around a third of participants significantly doubted themselves when giving information to families or felt that they were not experienced enough for their role. When considering the fear of 'the tap on the shoulder' asking them why they thought they were in the role, or the belief that one day someone will catch them out, this rose to almost half. This left almost half of participants finding themselves sometimes lying awake at night going over conversations they had that day worrying that they should have said something different.

Some of the respondents in the survey commented on why they felt that they experienced impostor syndrome. One of the core aspects raised was that to work in lactation support you need to have a thick skin in the face of the criticisms many of us face. As we know, and examined earlier in the chapter, many are all too quick to dismiss the role of lactation experts. This coupled with a lack of investment and funding in the role and it's easy to start thinking that your work is not valued.

> 'I often feel like my expertise isn't valued. I'm only with the Trust part time and some of my colleagues ignore my existence. I often find that my decisions are overridden and I have to be persistent in ensuring things get done. I'd say I was a pretty robust character but it's easy to start doubting yourself when it feels like so much is against you.' (IBCLC)

> 'It takes much strength not to feel defeated when so many think your role is not needed but I remind myself that they want me to feel this way and carry on.' (IBCLC)

This was intensified for those who came under fire on social media, which we will return to later on. For those who were active on social media and therefore more likely to be targets there was a feeling of being under continual criticism not necessarily for individual actions but more through the broader role of being a lactation supporter:

I am regularly told on social media that I am hurting women. It's hard not to start to doubt yourself.' (Peer supporter)

'Social media is mean and it takes courage not to internalise critical comments about ones worth as an LC [lactation consultant].' (IBCLC)

Another central issue impacting on feelings of impostor syndrome was the broader issue of so many women struggling to breastfeed in a society that doesn't support it. Many respondents in the survey talked about their limited ability to fix an issue despite so much good intention and guidance when there were so many other influences on a breastfeeding experience. It's difficult not to doubt yourself when faced with women who are still struggling or stop before they are ready despite everything you have tried to do.

'I think I cause my own issues sometimes with worrying that I'm not good enough in the role. I think it might be because although I do my best so many women I work with still struggle. I should be able to recognise by now that it's a result of other things going on in their lives which I'm pretty powerless to change. But even when I try to think like that the doubts often still creep in.' (Peer supporter)

'If someone could help me not blame myself when I spend time with a mother and she ends up stopping anyway that would be great.' (Peer supporter)

Was it something you said? Could you have done something differently? Are you not helping in the way you thought? These are all such common thoughts but are a result of the system rather than the care you are giving. Remember what we say to women – they do not fail to breastfeed instead they are failed by a system that fails to support them. By definition this affects your ability to support breastfeeding too. Every time a family member persuades a mother to let them give a bottle to 'help', someone criticises breastfeeding in public, or a council makes yet another cut... well that affects the challenges you have to overcome, often in a few hours per week in a church hall. Until the broader system is fixed there will always be casualties – and it appears that includes the wellbeing of those trying to pick up the pieces.

This links to one final reason you might doubt yourself – because the stakes are so high. Reflecting back on earlier sections on the impact of our own feeding experiences that many carry with them, coupled with that huge tendency to empathise and care, it can feel like the information and support you are giving a family can really make or break their feeding experience and mental health. Many of us remember that one person who gave us the support that made all the difference... and many of us carry not so great memories of the people who gave unhelpful (or frankly ludicrous) advice. Our brains lie awake at night asking us whether we will be the one person who manages to trigger that lightbulb moment in a mother, or the one that casts her further into darkness? It is that pressure which makes us start to doubt ourselves.

> 'It is all too easy to lie awake dissecting my interactions with parents. Did I help them? Did I help them ENOUGH?' (Breastfeeding counsellor)

> 'I don't think the doubts of 'did I do enough' ever go away no matter how long I am in this job.' (IBCLC – of 30+ years experience)

Although impostor thoughts were present across all groups in the survey, they were particularly prevalent amongst peer supporters - three quarters of whom were worried about being 'found out' and half worried about not being good enough in their role. This linked back to the issue of many peer supporters feeling that their training and qualifications were not recognised or underplayed by other health professionals in the area that they worked. Feeling like they didn't fit in or weren't useful deepened feelings of being an impostor. It also left over half feeling too scared to ask questions in case they were judged as not knowing enough.

'Sometimes this role terrifies me. I feel like everyone else knows what they're doing and what if I get it wrong and harm a mother's breastfeeding journey?' (Peer supporter)

'It feels like what I say carries too much weight. What if I get it wrong? It's not helped by having limited time. If I had more time to sit with mums rather than spending time recording everything I do maybe I wouldn't feel so worried about accidentally missing something.' (Peer supporter)

These feelings sometimes stopped peer supporters from progressing in their role or career, from fear that they would not be 'good enough' for other positions or anxiety about carrying additional responsibilities:

'I'd love to study for my IBCLC as parents tell me I'm a natural but then I think, me? I don't have any qualifications past my GCSES. What am I thinking?' (Peer supporter)

Bullying – the (lactating) elephant in the room

Unfortunately, we know that bullying at work is common in healthcare with research showing that approximately 20 – 25% of nurses and midwives experience bullying in the workplace from either peers or managers.[10] This is especially common amongst students. The phrase 'nurses eat their young' was first raised by Meissner, in 1986, to highlight the hierarchical bullying that can occur in the profession.[11] Students are bullied for their lack of experience coupled with their enthusiasm about making a difference. It is bizarre to witness within a profession which has caring for others at its heart.

Bullying in health care can take a number of forms but can include aspects such as humiliation, withholding of important information, blocking progress, spreading malicious information and exclusion from opportunities and events.[12] Unfortunately, it appears that lactation support is no different. Almost half of respondents in the survey said that they had experienced bullying behaviour from health care professionals that they worked with.

> *'Part of the reason I am now working privately is the bullying I experienced from senior consultants at the hospital. Their repeated attempts to undermine me destroyed my mental health.' (IBCLC, Neonatal nurse)*

> *'A parent made a complaint for supposedly pressuring her to breastfeed. My manager who sneered at breastfeeding policy took the opportunity to drag me through the complaints procedure for this.' (Health visitor)*

Sadly, a third felt that they had experienced bullying by other breastfeeding supporters. This was often more distressing than when it came from someone external.

> *'I was bullied out of my NHS role by another midwife in infant feeding. How can anyone in a caring role be so unkind?' (IBCLC, Midwife)*

> *'I have never been so distressed as when others in my field turned against me for doing something that they deemed unsuitable. One minute I was their respected peer and the next like something they'd trodden in.' (IBCLC)*

This also had a negative impact on those watching disagreements and infighting occur, especially when it caused divisions between once tight-knit groups. Over half stated that they had witnessed a lot of 'infighting' between breastfeeding supporters with three quarters finding disagreements distressing. The illogical nature of this amongst supporters who had, until this point, been able to see the complexity of a situation and trained to respond in a non-judgemental and caring way was highlighted by several in the survey:

'One of the most upsetting things I've seen in recent years - and I've seen it 3 times from the same organisation - is the denigration of another breastfeeding organisations work and workers. It benefits no-one.' (Breastfeeding counsellor)

'I feel sick when something kicks off and people who are supposed to be on the same side are trying to bring each other down. I lose all respect especially when they are supposedly stars in their field but are acting like children.' (Peer supporter)

Understandably, bullying can have significant mental health implications. Feelings of isolation, powerlessness and of being undermined are common, through to more serious issues of anxiety and depression.[13] Others can experience physical symptoms such as migraines, and insomnia, with chronic health issues exacerbated.[14] It is not uncommon for staff to leave a role or even the profession.[15] If bullying is public it can damage the reputation of a profession and affect patient / client wellbeing.[16] In similar roles such as midwifery and nursing, bullying is strongly linked to burnout.[17]

As you hopefully know deep down, bullying is rarely anything to do with the individual who is being bullied but instead stems from the insecurities or past experiences of the bully. In the healthcare workplace this can mean that many bullies feel powerless, or jealous and take that out on someone else. The concept of 'tall poppy syndrome' is rife in healthcare.[18] This is where promising young nurses, midwives and other healthcare students are systematically identified and attempts made to bring them down – simply for being so good at what they do.

Other research has shown that many bullies were themselves bullied earlier in their career. Theories have been built around how workplace bullying is so common in health care that students even learn how to do it, subconsciously or not, through their training and early careers with almost an expectation that one day they themselves will graduate to the position of bully.[19]

Bullying can take many forms including direct insults, blocking opportunities, and belittling in front of others. It can occur as a one-off event but typically is repetitive over time. One form of bullying which is more subtle, but can have far reaching impacts, is exclusion. In the survey, participants were asked if they had been made to feel that they don't fit in as a lactation professional or supporter specifically because of their background. For age, 15% felt that they were excluded or made to feel different because with this rising to 32% of those aged under 35 and 25% of those aged over 60. Both the younger and older group felt excluded because of their different experiences.

> 'I think some of the younger generation think I'm past it because I have grey hair. I still have a lot to   offer even if I'm not on Instagram.' (Breastfeeding counsellor)

> 'I'm a younger IBCLC and feel I'm looked down on because I don't have the experience. I don't have years of experience, but I have other skills and connections with mothers. Why can't we celebrate difference?' (IBCLC)

Education (18%) and socioeconomic background (12%) were felt to be another source of exclusion. In the free text comments this was raised predominantly in relation to having few qualifications or not living in an affluent area.

'I left school at 16 and had two children by the time I was twenty. I've got tattoos and hair that I change all the time. I don't live in the nice part of town and feel I'm different. I'm happy with who I am and know I support parents well - as they tell me - but I feel the other supporters don't accept me in the same way they do each other. It's not on purpose I don't think but it makes me feel different.' (Peer supporter)

'I'm very much working class and proud but it feels like other people come from a much more privileged background to me and it makes me subconscious.' (Peer supporter)

For ethnicity, 7% of participants felt that they were excluded because of their ethnicity; but of this group just 4% were from white backgrounds. Additionally, 6% of participants felt excluded because of their religion.

'I work in a neighbourhood full of Black and Brown mothers but I'm the only Black supporter. Why do people like me need support but not get to do the supporting role?' (Peer supporter)

'In relation to your question about feeling excluded based on who I am… I'm Jewish and although it's not deliberate I feel like I work in a very Christian or atheist centric location where my traditions are excluded. This makes it hard to attend some events and celebrations which makes me feel like I'm not properly included and thus accepted.' (IBCLC)

For LGBTQ status, 2% of the whole sample felt excluded but looking specifically at those who identified as LGBTQ, a third of this group felt that their sexuality and identity led to their exclusion.

'I don't feel so comfortable doing face-to-face work because I worry women will think I just want to look at their breasts since I'm gay, when really I just want to support them meet their breastfeeding goals.' (Breastfeeding counsellor)

'I'm outwardly very Queer and I think it makes some of my fellow supporters uncomfortable, even if it's just on a subconscious level.' (Peer supporter)

Finally, 12% of respondents felt that they were excluded due to their own feeding experiences, and 2% for not having their own children (or 74% of those without their own children).

'I am open about how I bottle fed one of my children and mixed fed the other. I think this gives me more understanding of different types of feeding experience but I have been judged for it by others who think I don't have enough breastfeeding experience and that the only right way to feed a baby is exclusive breastfeeding.' (Peer supporter)

'I'm often asked by mothers if I really understand because I don't have my own children. I do point out that the male obstetricians I've worked with never get asked this!' (Midwife)

There are two core intertwined issues at play here. First, the historic lack of diversity in lactation support, although slowly changing, still exists. The second is that even in 2019/2020 lactation supporters were *still* feeling excluded based on their background. Obviously, no one should *ever* be excluded, treated differently or looked down on for who they are, and this is unacceptable, regardless of whether individuals are being treated this way deliberately or through systemic ageism, classism, racism, ableism or homophobia. We do not always see who we exclude through our ways of working, even if the idea of exclusion would horrify us.

It is also at odds with what we, as lactation supporters, want to see - a world where more women are able to breastfeed, where fewer communities see it as unusual, and society values its worth. Although there are complex issues on breastfeeding rates and 'who breastfeeds', a lack of diversity in terms of who is working within lactation support is surely a key contributor. If women and families look at support networks and tend to see a certain type of person overrepresented, and those people do not match their background, culture and lifestyle, then will they feel fully comfortable accessing that support? I will return to this issue in the final chapter looking at a 'manifesto for change', signposting to many excellent diverse voices in this field who are leading change in this area.

In relation to supporters feeling excluded due to their own feeding experience, we know that this type of attitude exists but is thankfully increasingly in the minority. Personally, I would argue that our own personal experience of using formula, encountering breastfeeding challenges and experiencing grief at having to stop breastfeeding before we are ready adds insight, empathy and nuance to the support we offer. I know that many of those working in lactation support are brought here precisely by those very difficult experiences and that their practice benefits from that understanding.

Of course, and related to the point around exclusion of those without parenting experience, this doesn't mean that those who had more positive breastfeeding journeys cannot offer empathetic support. All of us have our own histories and broader life experiences that we bring to this field, across all different roles and responsibilities. But to exclude someone because they haven't exclusively breastfed for a certain duration is quite frankly ludicrous. It also links back to my previous point around ensuring that we, as supporters, represent the diversity of families that we deal with. Many families do use formula or stop breastfeeding before they are ready, either through choice or because their situation led them to that point. They gain comfort in knowing that many experts in this field have also had those experiences. I realise that if you're reading this book then I'm most likely preaching to the converted here, but tackling this persistent issue is of such importance on both an individual and societal level.

The role of social media

'I find I need to very carefully compartmentalise the politics around breastfeeding especially in media & social media. The anger and disrespect exert a huge toll on my emotional well-being if I do engage, so I have had to step away. I feel very sad I am not resilient enough to participate in this important space, but firstly I need to protect myself. Rescuing starfish is what I do, but I believe each individual starfish has huge value.' (Breastfeeding counsellor)

There are lots of arguments for using social media as part of lactation work. It's a useful way of connecting with colleagues and peers, in spreading public health information and supporting parents, and directly finding clients or bringing attention to a peer support group you are running. We know that parents find it a really useful way to receive breastfeeding support especially during the Covid-19 pandemic where many mothers turned to social media pages for advice and connection.[20,21] Numerous studies including from the US,[22,23] UK[24,25] and Australia[26] are now showing the value that mothers place on receiving support on these pages from a range of lactation professionals and volunteers, attributing this support to being able to breastfeed for longer.

Unfortunately, however, we all know that social media can also have a dark side. In more recent years attempts at damaging the reputation of professionals and preventing their work and progression have been common on social media with individuals or groups attacking prominent professionals and volunteers, often in a way that is hard to succinctly defend. It can be very difficult to respond to someone hurling untruths, mockery and abuse at you when you hold a professional position and have to be careful in any communication that you make (or indeed, would not want to respond in equal fashion). Nuance is also difficult to convey in 280 characters.

Sadly, this was reflected in survey responses with almost half of participants who were active on social media reported that they had been 'trolled' by others online e.g. receiving nasty comments, deliberate misinterpretation of their beliefs, and threats to their work or safety. Many of these trolling events came from those outside of breastfeeding support, or those who were actively working against breastfeeding support. Typically, the messaging at the heart of this trolling was untrue, unfair and harmful to those on its receiving end. While some could brush it off, over three quarters of those who had experienced this said that such comments made them feel anxious, unwell or affected their sleep. Conversely just 3% felt able to confidently ignore it.

> *'I get personal messages trolling saying that I only care about breastfeeding, not mothers' mental health etc. It is incredibly upsetting to see the same issues raised over and over and over again.' (Peer supporter)*

> *'I have lost sleep over social media attacks from those intent on obstructing breastfeeding support. It has made me incredibly unwell.' (Peer supporter)*

Some tried to stay away from social media arguments, but others felt that they had to step in, particularly if inaccurate or unhelpful information was being shared, with 40% stating that they spent a lot of time responding to breastfeeding debates because they wanted those watching to see correct information.

> *'I regularly promise that I'm leaving social media but it feels impossible to step back when there are so many untruths spreading.' (Breastfeeding counsellor)*

> *'I try to keep out of it until one of my friends is targeted and then it's war!' (Peer supporter)*

For some, the trolling and malicious interactions came from outside the lactation profession. Respondents across all groups had been accused of taking advantage of parents, brainwashing them or being overly judgemental and critical.

> *'I have received what I feel are threats to my livelihood but there was nothing that could be done.'* (IBCLC)

> *'Even though I know it's trolling and not fair, some comments written about me online have left me unable to sleep. It particularly hurts when they say I do not care about parents or am causing them to feel under pressure as it's categorically untrue and the opposite of who I am.'* (Breastfeeding counsellor)

Indeed, some found it particularly challenging when trolling comments were completely untrue. When comments were broad such as being 'evangelical about breastfeeding' they were easier to handle. Most supporters work with nuance in their work, placing families at the heart of their support. However, often attacks on social media undermined this, spreading misinformation.

> *'I've had public posts written about me saying I am anti formula and it isn't true. It's frustrating and hurtful.'* (Breastfeeding counsellor)

We know that personal attacks are a major issue on social media. Slurs around those considered to be 'fanatical' about breastfeeding are common,[27] with accusations thrown about that we are somehow turning breastfeeding into 'big business'.[28] We also know deep down that trying to change people's opinions online can be futile. If someone is angry / manipulative enough to troll or make sweeping generalisations or unfair criticism online, then it's highly unlikely that anything you say is going to change their view. Responding may be beneficial in terms of 'who is watching' but sometimes it's just easier to put down your phone and walk away.

A good measure I always go by is '*if I switch off social media, does this still matter?*' or in other words, does this matter to the people I work with, support and care for in real life? Sometimes it does, sometimes it doesn't. Sometimes disagreement is genuine (and important to reflect on) and sometimes it's a deliberate attempt to distract, enrage or alienate. Sometimes you have the energy to respond and try to correct misinformation, and sometimes you'd just rather walk away.

If you do get drawn into 'debates' on social media, do consider who is watching and the impact on your role and reputation. It is SO difficult when someone behind a nameless account, or who has little potential comeback from what they post online e.g. from an employer, decides to mock or antagonise you online. I bet there are many witty comebacks (or gifs) that you would like to use but it is worth stopping and thinking about how this might reflect on you. Sometimes a bit of humour can go a long way. Sometimes a rant is therapeutic for you and your readers. At other times we risk looking unprofessional, or even nasty in our responses, especially to an audience who might not fully see, nor understand, the nuance or background to the situation. It's worth considering how you would feel if this exchange was read out in court.

However, not all social media negativity is external to the profession. Others were negatively affected by watching fighting, criticism or falls outs between breastfeeding supporters online, with almost 80% stating that seeing such arguments break out about breastfeeding on social media really upset them.

> '*It saddens me greatly that my biggest critics have been from within.*' (IBCLC)

> '*I expected that it would be industry that came for me but plot twist, it's been my colleagues.*' (Infant feeding lead)

'One night I said something that was apparently wrong and all hell kicked off. I tried to explain what I meant and apologise but there was a small group of people who were determined to make me out to be a totally awful human being. On the one hand I could see what they were trying to do and it was about bringing me down a notch in their eyes but I still felt sick. I didn't sleep at all. It passed with time but I'll never forget it'. (Peer supporter)

As with 'face to face' arguments, many found witnessing arguments online between others in the profession stressful. Several commented that it was also distressing to watch as it made those involved, and by nature the lactation profession, appear unprofessional.

'I hate it when disagreements occur online and you're expected to pick a side. Why do we lose the ability to see nuance when it's our own?' (Breastfeeding counsellor)

'I wish our profession would act as if we were professionals and stop with the infighting. It's embarrassing to witness publicly and does us as an organisation no favors.' (Doula)

This is an extremely sensitive area to reflect on but one that is certainly worth doing. Many of us hold strong beliefs around topics such as sponsorship, bottles and other aspects of lactation support. Discussion, debate and reflection is good - necessary indeed. Sometimes behaviour or beliefs overstep a line that is unacceptable and almost all would consider to be too far to be solved through simple dialogue. But when we disagree with each other so publicly, what are the unintended consequences of that? What do our conflicts and put downs do to our core message of improving things for women, families and infant feeding? How do families who want a safe and reassuring space feel when they see the people they look to for support publicly fighting?

It was a sad element of the research findings that many respondents, some who asked not to be identified through their responses, had faced much harsher criticism from colleagues and peers than they had from the people they felt they were really fighting against. As one peer supporter pointed out, she felt that *'Some days the formula companies must be sat laughing at the profession tearing itself apart in a way the formula industry could never dream of.'*

Most disagreements are far more nuanced than a simple 'right or wrong' and the contexts and personal experiences that led to them are as diverse as the reasons why families we support stop breastfeeding. Again, this may be an obvious point to those of you reading this book, but I wish more broadly everyone could remember that ultimately, we are often fighting for the same thing, just in different ways.

Take home message: Disconnection is tough. Many of us feel lonely in our roles, or in conflict with others in our team which exacerbates a tendency to imposter syndrome and of doubting ourselves. It's hard enough to defend something we believe passionately in and field the external criticism. But when the criticism is from within it can hurt more. Let's always remember we're on the same side and who the real 'enemies' are. Oh, also remember that you will never win over everyone on social media, don't exhaust yourself trying!

Chapter 5

Financial pressures and privilege

'I just want to be able to book a room and offer mums a cup of tea. It's not exactly asking the world is it, given how much benefit we provide.' (Peer supporter)

Every occupation carries financial pressures, and the world of lactation is no different. From underfunding of services and a reliance on volunteers, through to critical views around charging for services, many in the survey found financial issues stressful for different reasons. This was intertwined with, and aggravated by, all the issues we've already discussed in this book - a lack of value for breastfeeding, patriarchal models of healthcare and a tendency to carry on giving regardless. Although some of the financial challenges overlap, I've broken these down into salaried, self-employed and voluntary posts (recognising that many hold multiple positions, alongside offering countless unpaid hours on top).

For those in salaried posts

Around a third of survey respondents were in a position where their infant feeding work was salaried, either in full or as part of their wider role. However even with this role over half did not feel confident that their post was secure long-term. Many had battled to secure their role in the first place with just a quarter saying that they found it easy to find a salaried paid role in breastfeeding support. Notably, when asked about whether they felt that their infant feeding related post was paid at an appropriate level, over half stated that they felt that they were asked to work at a pay grade lower than their experience.

'Much of my work is voluntary and the rest is underpaid!' (Breastfeeding counsellor)

'I feel I am underpaid for what I do but it took me 7 years to secure any type of paid post at all so complaining feels futile.' (Peer supporter)

'As a breastfeeding specialist I am aware that service provisions offered match that of senior feeding coordinators, however pay does not reflect this.' (Breastfeeding counsellor)

Despite having a paid role over two thirds of respondents felt that they could not fit their role into their paid hours. In theory and on paper they were paid to offer breastfeeding support but in reality, the number of families that needed support far outweighed this.

'I'm paid for 14 hours a week in this role. I work at least twice those hours. It's very difficult to say no to a mother who needs help because your hours are up. It's not that type of job and the pay isn't the real reason that I do it, but nevertheless it would be nice to be properly paid for what I do.' (Infant feeding lead).

'I would simply like someone to recognise all the additional hours that I work. I don't necessarily need to be paid for them, but I would like management to stop pretending that it's not happening.' (Midwife).

Others found that although supporting breastfeeding was part of their paid role, they were not allocated any time at all to fulfil this. Many ended up giving breastfeeding support in their free time. This obviously placed strain on the individual but also caused considerable frustration as they felt that the NHS was being propped up by their willingness to voluntarily support families.

'As a self-employed GP virtually ALL of my breastfeeding support is done unpaid. I want to become an IBCLC but at present I can't afford the unpaid time off, locum fees or the cost of education.' (GP).

'I was asked to act up as infant feeding lead for our area while my colleague was on long term sick leave but wasn't given any additional time to do it. It was suggested that because I was already working with families that I was somehow already doing the role. I worked myself into the ground before holding up my hands and saying I can't do this. It's not something that can be squeezed around the edges!' (Health visitor).

This became problematic when difficult cases arose. Either professionals did not have time to adequately address the problem, or in some cases it caused significant difficulties if things went wrong.

'I hate having to walk away from a mother because I have no time left. But I have a family to support so I can only offer a few hours a week. That's often fine and I feel like I'm doing my bit but it's horrible when I have to leave to get to my job and a mother is fighting back the tears with a baby who won't latch and I can't stay.' (Breastfeeding counsellor)

'I had a case where I was trying to offer support for a mother as part of a social media group but she didn't give full details of how much weight her baby had lost. I did tell her that she really needed someone to see her baby face to face but had encouraged her to keep breastfeeding based on the information she had given me. The baby was admitted with dehydration and this caused all manner of complications because it was suggested that I was doing this unpaid and didn't have the support of my line manager or even legal protection through work. It was sorted in the end but it was deeply stressful'. (Midwife)

Others faced challenges because although their role was funded, there were not additional funds for aspects of their role that were vital to delivering a good service. This included a lack of additional staffing and resources, but more broadly it included elements such as not being able to hire venues for peer support because there was simply no budget in place. Although a local hall hire may only cost a small amount it was a major barrier to delivering a service with many, peer supporters in particular, scrabbling around to find free venues which then were often affected by size or timing issues.

> *'Our service relies on peer supporters but our area made the decision to defund peer supporter training. Make it make sense?' (Health visitor)*

> *'All grant funding has been cut, NHS stopped funding it even though it addresses one of their priorities which isn't being met in other ways.' (Breastfeeding counsellor)*

For those self-employed

Those who were self-employed in the survey were typically working in private practice as IBCLCs. Some had additional paid work in other roles, many of which were not connected directly to lactation support. Only a minority were in part-time health professional roles and working in private practice alongside this. This may well be linked as one survey respondent noted:

> *'I'm employed as a midwife part time, and it was suggested to me that working as a lactation consultant outside of work was a conflict of interest although how exactly I'm not sure. The irony is that they won't pay me to offer lactation consultant level support as part of my role, saying that there's no funding for that.' (Midwife)*

Being self-employed offered its own challenges, predominantly due to a continual battle to make the work profitable. Only 15% of those who were self-employed in the survey agreed with the statement that *'I make enough money from my breastfeeding work for it to be a profitable, well paid position'*. Many also disliked the uncertainty of not having a secure stream of income with two thirds of survey respondents finding it stressful having to look for the next 'customer'. Indeed, as two IBCLCs noted:

'I'd like to be able to make a living by offering breastfeeding support (to not need a "day job").' (IBCLC)

'I'd like to be able to make a living and provide (some) services for free or at lower cost.' (IBCLC)

This was made worse by seemingly illogical peaks and troughs in demand for support which many in the survey raised as a considerable challenge to both earning a sufficient wage in other roles and planning support. If some weeks demand is high, how do you offer that support if you are committed to another part time role? And what do you do in the weeks where lactation enquiries are low or absent but you cannot increase your hours in your other job?

'Sometimes I go for weeks without earning enough to even break even with my costs and then ten requests come in at once and I have to turn work away because they are all urgent and there are only so many families I can support at the same time.' (IBCLC).

'It would help if I had a more steady flow of families using my services.' (Breastfeeding counsellor)

This led to a feeling amongst some practitioners that they would never be able to fully scale their business because they were reliant on having to earn enough money in another role. To them it felt that working as an IBCLC, or other private practitioner, was limited to those with savings or few outgoings, a supportive partner or a small window when already at home caring for small children (which obviously created its own pressures). This of course skewed the demographics of who was able to be offering services:

'I can't afford to get my practice off the ground. If I was rich then we could suck up my start-up costs or lean weeks but I'm stuck in a circle where I can't afford to give up my job but my job also means I can't grow.' (IBCLC)

'We have a lack of diversity in lactation care because of the financial barriers to training and starting up.' (IBCLC)

Some found always having to charge for their services challenging because they felt distressed when they knew that parents couldn't afford them. In total 86% of respondents struggled with this element, with some noting that they tried to provide some free or reduced cost support where possible. Almost all respondents worried that it was those who needed the support most who often could not afford it.

'I really struggle to charge people sometimes and often find myself thinking about whether I should lower my prices or give things away for free. But my training cost a lot of money and I have bills to pay. I have to charge for what I do but I feel guilty.' (IBCLC).

'I know a particular demographic accesses my services and the conspicuous absence of who is not there eats away at me. I offer limited free support without broadcasting this out of fear it will upset those paying.' (IBCLC)

Although some were able to account for this in other ways, through pricing structures or exchanging other skills, two thirds of respondents noted that they regularly gave their time away for free because parents could not afford to pay for the support they desperately needed.

'My standard prices now include a small amount to cover a limited amount of emergency support for families who really need it but can't afford it.' (IBCLC)

> *'I promise myself I'm going to stop offering free support but then a mother gets in contact with a pressing problem but no means to pay my full costs. What am I meant to do? Walk away? In what conscience?'* (IBCLC)

However, this generosity and flexibility could be a double-edged sword. Almost half of survey respondents felt that this meant that some families took advantage of them, often when they could have paid but had only wanted free advice. This was a broad issue with 80% of those who completed the survey feeling frustrated at people's expectations that you would provide support for free, even when individuals could afford it.

Many a social media inbox was overflowing with 'quick questions' which a) certainly would often not be quick to answer and b) would take more than the hours available in a day to answer them all and c) are a legal and ethical minefield, because once you have provided 'advice', whether free or charged, you have entered into a working relationship, and you then have a duty of care to that person. If, based on incomplete assessment or anything else, that advice turns out to be erroneous, you can still be held accountable.

> *'One individual asked for support with a complex issue. When I explained that I would need to see her and that this was my pricing structure she got angry and accused me of ripping her off when she was in pain. I felt terrible but I couldn't help her without taking a full history and going to see her. I can't be expected to do that for free?'* (IBCLC).

> *'I don't ask for proof of low income for my discounted or free sessions as that is demeaning. It works on mutual trust and respect but sometimes I have a feeling a parent could pay me but that they are choosing not to. It hurts.'* (IBCLC).

Others faced criticism when they did have a fair pricing structure for their work and were accused of 'profiting' from breastfeeding or having extortionate rates. Some critics felt that lactation professionals overcharged or should not even be charging for their time or expertise at all. The experience of being criticised for 'profiting' from families has arisen in research, with an unfair suggestion that the field is over medicalising breastfeeding in order to profit from it.[1] This experience was common in the survey:

'I've seen posts accusing me of making money from vulnerable families and it feels so unfair. Why shouldn't I make money from my knowledge and experience? Why is it ok for a mechanic to charge me hundreds of pounds to fix my car but me not to charge to fix something that is often more important?' (IBCLC).

'Some other peer supporters got funny with me when I started getting some pay for my role. I don't know if it was jealousy or a genuine belief we should give our time for free but I'm giving up a lot of time and am good at what I do. Why shouldn't I get paid?' (Peer supporter)

Unfortunately, pay issues are sometimes ignited by a small group of unqualified individuals posing as experts at an extortionate cost. Despite a very different ethos and way of working, the whole field ends up getting tarnished with the same brush. Some reflected on this:

'I've seen people with no qualifications set themselves up as feeding experts or sleep trainers and charge a small fortune for their support. They often cause more problems - the number who end up coming to see me after receiving poor support from them and then not being able to afford my support drives me crackers.' (IBCLC)

Those working in management positions within organisations, or even in infant feeding research related posts also faced this criticism. Often these posts are fairly well paid compared to the average wage, but this is because they carry with them considerable responsibility, or reflect the extensive training and experience that has led to an individual having this role.

> 'I hold an executive role in an infant feeding related organisation which I do not wish to disclose due to likely backlash. I have received criticism directly to my face and have been made aware of discontent in our organisation and others because I am paid. My post is managerial and has considerable pressures and this attitude frustrates me deeply.' (Charity role)

> 'I was accused of exploiting families with my research because I am in a well paid post. I am not tenured and do not have job security but it hurt most of all because I chose this field because I think they will benefit marginalised communities, not myself. My colleagues in other fields do not face these accusations.' (Peer supporter, Researcher)

Indeed, this strange concept of accusing lactation supporters of profiting from families is often seen on social media despite its absurdity. We may respond by joking about our 'billions from breastfeeding' but in all honesty, would this happen for any other area of health? Do we accuse those working for the police as profiting from crime? Physiotherapists as profiting from unfortunate incidents on the football pitch? Michelin star restaurant owners overpricing their exquisite food compared to the local café? Why shouldn't experts be paid for their knowledge and time? There are also considerable time and financial costs involved in training at any level in lactation support including professional updates, travel, and all the work that is done outside of an appointment time once qualified. Quite rightly, costs need to include this.

Again, the anger and frustration that many face is misplaced. We *shouldn't* have to pay for private health care, not least for infant feeding support. It should be accessible, plentiful and practitioners well paid. Instead, because the government fails to value breastfeeding enough to invest sufficiently in different lactation support roles, the onus falls on communities to deliver these services. To allow those providing it the chance to eat and keep a roof over their heads they have to charge. And those charges should reflect the expertise, training and experience that went into achieving that role. Lawyers and tradesmen don't tend to flinch at fairly pricing their work, so why should lactation supporters be any different?

For those in voluntary positions

Most of those working in voluntary positions were working in a peer support capacity. The combination of a lack of pay and qualifications that were sometimes perceived as 'less than' rather than 'different' led to almost three quarters of peer supporters feeling concerned that they were looked down on by some paid professionals. The key word here is obviously 'some' with a number of peer supporters clarifying in their responses that often it was those working outside of lactation but who they came into contact with in their role who dismissed their worth.

> *'Here in [redacted], we are regularly told how important us volunteers are, how we save so much money for the NHS, how the families we deal with really appreciate us. Yet we never see any reward. The NHS wouldn't even pay for the postage of Christmas cards our peer support coordinator bought for us. I know the NHS is struggling financially, but if we are saving so much money with our volunteering, shouldn't we have something to show thanks, even a postage stamp? If it wasn't for the support of [redacted] and her team, who are so supportive of what we do, I would not still be doing what I'm doing. I don't believe those higher up within the NHS understand what we do, or appreciate us. It's as if they forget we are doing this in our own time. I give up a morning a week, to volunteer; I could be at work, earning money. I'm not the only one who feels this way.'*
> *(Peer supporter)*

Two thirds of volunteers also felt that the work they did was not valued because they were not paid. This was deeply ironic given that earlier on in the survey, when exploring service funding and cuts, many respondents felt that the system was propped up by the good will of volunteers, including their additional labour over and above their salaried hours. Indeed, a staggering 89% agreed with the statement that *'breastfeeding support in my area relies heavily on volunteers'*. It is unsurprising that many end up feeling like 'Schrödinger's peer supporter' – both indispensable and dispensable at the same time.

> *'I like volunteering and do not need to be paid from a financial perspective. I do however need to feel valued and that sadly is missing right now.'* (Peer supporter)

Others really struggled with boundaries. Although those volunteering were obviously expecting to provide some support for free, many felt that a few people would take advantage of this by asking for detailed support outside of volunteering hours

> *'I love helping at peer support group but sometimes local families track me down online asking for more information and it's just too much. I feel under pressure to help but sometimes just have to say can you come to group and we can help you there.'* (Peer supporter)

Notably however not all of those in voluntary positions wanted a paid role. Around two thirds stated that they would love a paid role but could not find one, and a third were content to carry on working in a volunteer capacity. Those who did not want a paid role typically wanted to give their time back to the communities that supported them, or were happy to spend time helping others.

> *'I feel that if I am not paid then I am working on my own terms and I prefer that.'* (Peer supporter)

People volunteer for many reasons and not everyone wants to be paid for every role they have. This includes factors linked to the volunteering experience (i.e. sense of giving back, altruism, being part of a positive system of change) but also changes to roles when payment is involved. For example, paid roles often carry more bureaucracy and paperwork, and earnings can impact upon other finances. Ultimately it can feel like the relationship between volunteer and service user, or the nature of the work has changed when money is involved.

Expectations and perceived power relations and hierarchies can all be subtly different. Notably, research with paid peer supporters found that most came into the role through altruism and simply wanted to help. However, when they took on 'official' roles (that could still be unpaid) they were then faced with procedures and paperwork which took their time away from supporting mothers. They then felt as if they had to meet targets and felt the pressure of accountability.[2]

Training and development challenges

Aside from pay and work opportunities, another closely related issue was the financial pressures of training in the first place. As noted above, financial privilege was felt to determine who could afford to set up in private practice or indeed who could go without payment and volunteer in roles. It also presented a barrier to those wanting to undertake further training, qualify as an IBCLC or to keep up with professional development costs. Overall, 70% of self-employed respondents found the cost of training or keeping up to date a big worry, with two thirds also struggling to find the time for continued development.

> 'I qualified for my IBCLC award 5 years ago but am already worrying about accessing sufficient credits to maintain and of course update my knowledge. I do not earn enough to be able to afford training days or conferences away from home. There needs to be flexibility for people like me.' (IBCLC).

'We are a low-income household and the cost of CERP certified study is a strain on our budget. Keeping up to date is no doubt essential but I would like to be able to evidence it in different low or no cost ways.' (IBCLC)

Training and development costs were more of a mixed issue for those working in voluntary roles. Some noted that they received their initial training and updates for free and were grateful for that opportunity. Naturally, if you want people to volunteer for your organisation, typically in unpaid posts, then you need to provide this opportunity. However, research suggests that it may bizarrely lead to animosity from those in more skilled positions because they cannot access so many training and development opportunities.

For example, one study highlighted how other healthcare professionals can feel undervalued if considerable funding and training is offered to peer supporters. Some find themselves in the position of having less breastfeeding specific training and updates than volunteers did.[3] Yet again, this is a casualty of a system that does not value and invest in infant feeding and instead results in those within the system end up turning on each other.

Access to training outside of their day-to-day role was often prohibitive for volunteers. Overall, 92% of those in voluntary positions found the cost of training or keeping up to date a big worry, with 82% agreeing that they could not afford to train for further qualifications such as taking the IBCLC exam because they were not paid.

'I can just about afford to sit the IBCLC exam but am not confident that I would then be able to commit to all the additional training needed to keep my registration.' (Breastfeeding counsellor)

Even some paid professionals found that system prohibitive due to cost and a lack of support. Many managers refused to support requests for relevant training or to sit examinations, even though they would benefit the workplace too. This comes back to organisations not valuing breastfeeding or the impact it can have:

'I want to train for my IBCLC exam but I can't afford it especially with the updates I would have to pay for to maintain registration. I know I have the knowledge and the experience but my manager has refused a request for funding despite the fact that they would benefit. It messes with my head.' (Infant feeding lead).

'In the past we were funded to go on study days such as the Baby Friendly conference and it meant so much to us to have that opportunity but this was reduced to a few chosen colleagues and then removed entirely.' (Infant feeding lead).

Others struggled with having one defined qualification for becoming an IBCLC, specifically in relation to training pathways and the process of keeping up to date. Amongst these respondents, many felt that the system excluded them and kept one type of practitioner more likely to be able to train and practice (this included in terms of socioeconomic background and neurodiversity).

'The IBCLC qualification system is prohibitive. It feels like there is one pathway and they hold all the power. It needs an overhaul that reflects people's different circumstances.' (Breastfeeding counsellor).

'I feel like I don't fit the mould for who gets to train as an IBCLC. I have ADHD and Autism and find traditional study difficult alongside attending big conferences. I feel different which to me should be the reason I train but in reality is keeping me from doing so.' (Peer supporter)

Our recent research led by Dr Aimee Grant highlighted that many Autistic women struggle with finding sensitive breastfeeding support.[4] This makes the responses highlighting the challenges that neurodiverse supporters additionally face even more pertinent. Are we compounding the issue by placing limits on those with lived experience of neurodiversity and breastfeeding? For example, the pandemic has increased access to training opportunities for many who feel uncomfortable travelling or being in large groups (or who prefer to and learn best in their own style at home). Although many value in person conferences restarting, we must make sure we don't lose sight of those who learn best in other ways, or shut off access to those who cannot, or prefer not to travel.

Take home message: Never forget your worth whether you receive financial payment or not. Never doubt yourself in charging fairly for your services - you deserve to be paid for your time and expertise. Ignore the annoying critics on social media. And if you're a manager reading this, or in a position where you can show those who give their time (for free or not) that they are valued, and haven't told everyone today that they're brilliant, please tell them (and some more)!

Chapter 6

The impact of the Covid-19 pandemic

The Covid-19 pandemic had far reaching consequences across all walks of life. People were affected in a multitude of ways, whether through the direct impact of the virus upon their health or the containment measures put in place to try to control the virus. I wrote more broadly about the impacts of the pandemic upon pregnancy, birth and postnatal care in my book 'Covid Babies', but in this chapter I want to particularly hone in upon the impacts of the pandemic for those doing the caring work.

Research has highlighted how those working in perinatal care were affected in a multitude of ways including experiencing distress due to having to change their care, an increase in workload and concerns for their own safety.[1] I know of no published research specifically focusing on the experiences of lactation supporters during that time despite, as noted earlier, awareness of this issue being raised by several who were concerned at the growing pressures. This is against a backdrop of plentiful evidence of how greatly mothers and families valued and appreciated the support, and how much those working in breastfeeding support stepped up to carry on delivering as much support as possible.[2,3]

As described in the introduction, I repeated a short version of the survey specifically in relation to burnout questions during the first Covid-19 pandemic lockdown from May - June 2020. At this point many countries were still in a strict lockdown. In the UK, for example, schools started to slowly open towards the start of June, but non-essential shops were still closed until mid-June. Other countries followed different timelines but for most at this time working and care practices were disrupted.

We know that infant feeding experiences were affected by the pandemic. Although some mothers reported some benefits due to a slower pace of life, fewer visitors, and more opportunity to spend time together as a new family, others struggled to access the support that they needed.[4,5] This was not helped by inaccurate messaging particularly on social media at the start of the pandemic concerning the safety of breastfeeding, expressing and storing milk. Research from around the world identified maternal concerns around safety, with some stopping breastfeeding due to this.[4,6,7] Evidence later emerged that mothers who were exposed to Covid-19 or who received the Covid-19 vaccination produced antibodies in their breast milk which may protect their baby.[8] However, despite supportive messages from the World Health Organisation that breastfeeding was safe and to be encouraged, it still caused significant distress.[9]

Research has examined how changes to care affected other healthcare professionals. For example, the 'State of Health Visiting in England' report for 2020 explored the experiences of 862 Health Visitors in England who had cared for families during the pandemic.[10] It found that 75% of health visitors who took part reported increased stress and 70% longer working hours. Overall, 69% felt worried, tense and anxious, 51% reported that their sleep was affected and 40% were experiencing low mood due to work related stress. In another study with 758 nurses and midwives in Turkey, two thirds were feeling anxious and uncertain, with almost half feeling that they needed psychological support. In fact, 12% were so distressed by the situation that they wanted to leave.[11]

So what about lactation supporters? In the second stage of my survey 520 lactation professionals and volunteers took part, from countries around the world, again as described in the introduction. For the personal burnout scale 72% of survey respondents were considered to have moderate or above levels of personal burnout compared to 60% before the pandemic. Meanwhile 28% had high levels compared to 23% in the pre-pandemic survey.

In terms of the proportion who felt these emotions or symptoms 'Always or often' over the last two weeks:

- Feeling tired: 79%
- Feeling physically exhausted: 58%
- Feeling emotionally exhausted: 94%
- Feeling that you can't take it anymore: 57%
- Feeling worn out: 95%
- Feeling weak and susceptible to illness: 61%

For the work-related burnout scale 71% of respondents were considered to have moderate or above levels of personal burnout (up from 59% pre pandemic) with 27% experiencing high levels (up from 19% pre pandemic). In terms of the proportion who felt these emotions or symptoms 'Always or often' over the last two weeks:

- Feeling that work is emotionally exhausting: 80%
- Feeling burnt out because of work: 52%
- Feeling frustrated by work: 81%
- Feeling worn out at the end of the working day: 97%
- Feeling exhausted in the morning at the thought of another day at work: 72%
- Feeling that every working hour is tiring: 54%
- Feeling enough energy for family and friends during leisure time: 54%

Of course, some of these feelings would have been intensified by the general impact of living through a global pandemic and worrying about the health of family and others - with wall-to-wall media coverage heightening that anxiety. Increased emotional and practical care loads of supporting vulnerable family and home schooling would have increased pressure. However, participant reflections suggested that it was also the impact of trying to care for families through this period in relation to changes to care.

'The pandemic sees us in a situation where the pressure to breastfeed is heightened but the support is even less available. It's disastrous and depressing knowing you have the knowledge to help but not the platform to do it because you can, no longer attend groups.' (Peer supporter)

A lack of face-to-face care was evident across postnatal care. In the State of the Nation Health Visiting in the UK only 79% of health visitors were able to offer all families a new birth visit and 67% a 6 – 8 week check. Some of these appointments were conducted by community nursery nurses or family support workers instead, which went against Public Health England guidance. Some of these checks were also completed over phone or video call.[10] In another study led by University College London with 740 Health visitors in England, only 47% conducted face to face new birth visits.[12] In an Irish study new mothers talked about how visits were often split. Some aspects of a visit were conducted over the phone, with mothers then being seen face to face for physical checks.[13] The ramifications of this were that mothers needed even greater support from other sources because they were less able to access it as part of postnatal care.

This notably was affected in part by redeployment in the UK during the first lockdown. Many midwives and health visitors were redeployed from community posts back into hospital roles, obviously leaving fewer professionals available to help new mothers. Overall, 66% of local authorities in England redeployed at least one member of the health visiting team, with 11% redeploying 25% or more. This meant that health visitor caseloads increased at a time where family needs also increased.[12] The impact of this was keenly felt in the survey.

'The NHS service I work for was completely suspended during the pandemic. We've been left sat at home or redeployed into inappropriate roles whilst mums & babies struggle and suffer.' (Peer supporter)

'I'm particularly frustrated by our Tongue Tie Service being abolished and our dedicated Breastfeeding Midwives being pulled to be 'frontline' midwives when staffing isn't short currently. Also our Special Care Baby Unit has a two hour visiting time limit per day for Mums which has had a tremendous impact on their Mental Health, I think now they are slightly more adaptive for Breastfeeding Mums but that's been difficult.' (Infant feeding support worker)

Video calls played a central role in all our communications during the pandemic, not least breastfeeding support. Organisations reacted rapidly to this, and mothers who accessed support in this way valued the practical and emotional support that it brought.[2,3] Response to this new approach was mixed amongst participants in the survey. Some found it actually enhanced their care and allowed them to support *more* mothers and families.

'Getting to grips with providing new-style 'lockdown' services has been a rollercoaster. intense, exhausting, overwhelming, exciting. I feel like I have found my feet a bit now, though, and am actually loving this new way of working. I'm reaching far more families than before, having moved my support work online rather than purely having face-to-face groups. I'm tired, but reinvigorated.' (IBCLC)

'One silver lining is that our weekly breastfeeding Zoom meeting is better attended than previous support groups which is satisfying.' (Breastfeeding counsellor)

Indeed, some mothers very much valued online support. In our study exploring the support offered by breastfeeding charities in the UK, 86% of mothers who completed a survey found one to one video calls useful, 84% social media posts useful, 75% group video calls useful and 70% text messages useful. Overall, 98% agreed that online support was useful during the pandemic with 81% wanting it to remain as an option when face to face meeting was possible again, to complement alongside face-to-face support.[2] However, others in the survey were concerned about those who were not able to access this method of communication so well due to deprivation and communication issues.

> *'I'm taking lots of calls but only from certain families. I'm worried about who I'm not seeing through this new way of working.' (IBCLC)*

> *'Video works well for some but sometimes you need to be in the room to really read what's going on.' (IBCLC)*

Undeniably, a move to video calls to provide support is often not equitable. Although some parents were satisfied with, or even preferred, increased access to video and phone call support during the pandemic, others struggled. Video calls also require the use of technology and a stable internet connection which pushes families from more deprived backgrounds, or those in remote areas with no access to high-speed broadband, further into disadvantage. Indeed, this digital divide was also clear in our breastfeeding research. Mothers who had high speed wi-fi and decent devices to access the internet on were less likely to stop breastfeeding than those who struggled to access online support.[4]

In another study with nurses working at a Maternal, Infant, and Early Childhood Home Visiting service in Florida found that whilst video calls worked well with some families, it raised a number of issues around internet connectivity, cost and a lack of suitable devices. Many ended up switching off video to get a better connection but this of course meant that all visual connection was lost, reducing emotional connection and meaning that nurses could not assess parent – infant interactions. Other families simply did not have the digital skills to conduct video calls in an effective way.[14]

Many in the survey were worried that they could not offer support to families in the same way over video call. It was clear that breastfeeding support is about more than simply offering information that could be conveyed across a screen but encompasses a holistic approach around wellbeing and checking in on parents.

'Video calls are great, but I worry we are missing signs of postnatal depression or troubles that would usually come out over a cup of tea at group.' (Breastfeeding counsellor)

'It breaks my heart not to be able to offer in person support. I know I am not offering the gold standard of care over conference call that I usually do.' (IBCLC)

This anxiety about the increased needs of parents during a time where support is less available has been highlighted by the Institute of Health Visiting. The 'State of Health Visiting in England' report for 2020 found that compared to two years ago over 80% of health visitors who took part felt that there had been an increase in domestic violence, poverty and perinatal mental illness during the pandemic. This was echoed in the UCL survey which found that almost all health visitors in the survey were worried about domestic abuse, safeguarding and parental mental health during the pandemic.[12]

Although phone calls can be useful in supporting some aspects of health care, particularly for simple queries, their impact upon more complex issues is often more negative. Understandably, individuals can often be reluctant to talk about intimate or personal issues such as mental health or domestic violence over the phone. When compared with face-to-face support, contacts are typically shorter, with less disclosure of information when conducted over the phone.[15]

This was echoed in research during the pandemic. One interview study with pregnant and new mothers highlighted how many felt they couldn't disclose personal information over the phone, particularly in relation to their mental health. Others missed the reassurance of someone seeing their baby face to face.[16] Another study in the US found that when women tried to describe physical issues over the phone, such as episiotomy or wound pain, their symptoms were often missed or misinterpreted.[17]

It was clearly evident in survey responses that many lactation supporters were experiencing significant overwhelm at changes to care. They were not just a bit frustrated or disappointed but struggling to manage their distress at having to care for families so differently. The trauma that many experienced in relation to those they were trying to support receiving poor care was clear:

> 'It's been frustrating during covid how the already weak system for new mums has completely fallen apart. Mums are told they can't have any help with breastfeeding and call us weeks later to relactate. It is emotionally hard to take on so many mums grief over lack of support and guilt at not feeding and their struggles with relactation. I am coping with this fine on a personal level as have good supervision in my organisation but I can't fix the system and that is where it gets frustrating.' (Peer supporter)

> 'Not being able to help a mother who is stopping breastfeeding is awful at the best of times but knowing it may have been different for her without these restrictions is awful. It's traumatic I would say and I'm struggling to process the logic of it.' (Breastfeeding counsellor)

This brings us back to the concept of vicarious trauma caused by being unable to support mothers effectively and seeing their breastfeeding journey damaged as a result. The concept of 'moral injury' has been raised in relation to other healthcare professionals working during the pandemic and it is clearly also relevant to the lactation profession. Moral injury occurs when health professionals are unable to care for parents in the way that they have been trained to, prefer and typically do so. Restrictions and regulations during the pandemic meant that certain aspects or ways of caring (such as face to face visits, group meet ups and physical touch and reassurance) were altered or withdrawn.

Research has highlighted how maternity care staff were at risk of moral injury simply due to being aware of changes to services in a way that first time parents were not, and additionally experiencing distress at knowing they were not caring for parents in an optimal way.[18] This was echoed in a study with doulas, many of whom were prevented from supporting parents during labour due to hospital restrictions. Many felt frustration and anxiety knowing that they could not care for their clients in the same way, and knowing what parents were missing out on.[19] Others felt dismissed and undervalued as they knew that they could play an important role in supporting parents and easing pressure on the health service, yet were unable to do so.[20]

Another distressing aspect was having to change the way that care was delivered even when it could be face to face. In the survey some lactation supporters described how even when they could do face to face visits they were unable to engage with mothers in the same way.

'We can do home visits where necessary but are told to limit them, keep them as short as possible and maintain our distance. It's just not the same and it's horrible when a mother is clearly distressed and needs someone to sit and listen.' (Health visitor)

'We call them in person visits but I don't feel they really are. I may be physically there across the room but that's not the same as truly being with woman.' (IBCLC).

The requirement to socially distance has been recognised as a significant challenge that many healthcare practitioners found distressing. One study with midwives explored how many felt that care was 'dehumanised' and although they tried to convey emotion and support using their eyes and body language, many missed being able to reach out, touch and comfort a mother.[21] Another global study with 127 midwives, obstetricians and other healthcare workers from 71 countries highlighted how many were instructed to carry out physical checks as quickly as possible, which felt brusque and insensitive when carrying out intimate examinations which are improved by reassurance and gentle care. Many talked about how this need to create physical distance resulted in emotional distance between caregiver and mother.[22]

Working with PPE was also distressing for some in positions where face to face care was possible. This included the discomfort and additional time that PPE caused but also how it created a barrier between supporter and mother, especially when trying to have conversations about emotional wellbeing.

'The wearing of PPE whilst having involved conversations with mums both about their feelings as well as explaining 'mechanical' aspects of breastfeeding are exhausting - not to forget the anxiety of catching the virus.' (Specialist breastfeeding supporter)

'I am hands on in my practice in relation to providing emotional support and positive body language (not with the baby). It's hard to try to convey this trussed up in protective clothing and a mask - but necessary I guess.' (IBCLC)

Indeed, research with other healthcare professionals found that PPE was a challenge for many during the pandemic, particularly in the warmer months. It added further time to any shift and some reported having to take more breaks away from parents as they were overwhelmed by the discomfort.[21] Changes to cleaning routines also meant that less time was spent supporting parents. In some hospitals it also led to changes in how women could be supported, particularly during labour.[22]

Others felt overwhelmed by the enormity of the broader situation and had cut down on how much breastfeeding support work they were doing due to other pressures at home such as home schooling, care or concern for their own safety. Even then providing support could still feel like too much.

'My breastfeeding workload has drastically reduced to about 1/8 of my usual, but even that feels like too much right now. Dreading opening my emails every day.' (IBCLC)

'I'm trying to limit support to the evenings when my children are in bed or occupied but I'm struggling to cope as am so exhausted.' (IBCLC)

We know from data that has now been collected from across the pandemic that women (on average) bore the brunt of the additional caring responsibilities that the pandemic caused, whether that was through supporting family, home schooling or additional household chores that having a family home caused. Research from the early weeks of the pandemic and that first lockdown showed that on average working mothers' hours were significantly reduced but working fathers showed little difference.[23]

A further concern particularly for those who were self-employed was contracting the virus and not being able to work. This would mean losing income but also letting families down.

'I am terrified of becoming too sick to work or having long lasting complications. Who would care for the families I support?' (IBCLC)

'I am worried about what happens if I get sick. Or worse still, what if I made a new mom sick? I'm trying to balance my anxieties with caution but it's overwhelming.' (IBCLC)

These anxieties were evident in research examining other healthcare professionals' concerns. Many were worried at the implications of contracting the virus including personal health concerns, but also the impact of not being able to work and the impact upon their colleagues if they were unable to attend work. In one study with midwives in the UK, many described feeling shock and concern for themselves if a woman they were caring for tested positive, whilst at the same time as feeling anxiety, concern and empathy for what this would mean for the mother and her birth and postnatal experience.[21]

Likewise, would a mother's breastfeeding care be affected if she became unwell? Would she be able to receive the support she needed, or feel like she should stop? In our research with breastfeeding women we found that 6% of mothers who had stopped breastfeeding did so because they had symptoms of Covid-19. It is possible that they felt too unwell to care for their baby, but we also found that 20% of women were worried about the safety of breastfeeding if they were infected with Covid-19.[4]

However, turning back to the core focus for many - families. For the scale, items specifically around supporting families showed much less of a difference. Overall, just 10% were experiencing moderate to high levels of burnout here (up from 8%) with just 2% showing high symptoms (up from 1% - which I'm sure dodgy headline writers would describe as DOUBLING). For specific items, the proportion of supporters who felt emotions 'Always or often' over the last two weeks was:

- Finding it hard to work with families: 7%
- Finding it frustrating to work with families: 5%
- Drained of energy by working with families: 13%
- Feeling that they give more back than you when working with families: 6%
- Tired of working with families: 5%
- Wondering how long they will be able to continue working with families: 15%

Interesting, isn't it? It appears that no matter how much the stress is dialled up, the work at the core of your role in supporting families doesn't feel that much more stressful. Again, it is everything that surrounds it that is the issue and not the central caring work. Finally, it was also evident that not everyone who responded felt that the pandemic had made them feel more stressed or overwhelmed. For some, just like with some parents, changes to everyday life and working arrangements felt positive, or enabled positives to emerge.

> *'I'm actually preferring working this way. There is less travel or stressing and it feels more manageable. Parents seem happy with what I'm offering too.' (IBCLC)*

> *'I'm an introvert and kinda liking this way of working. I'm reaching more families and it feels more relaxed.' (IBCLC).*

Take home message: You've just lived and worked through a pandemic. Be kinder to yourself. Even if you and your family have their health, this doesn't mean that it wasn't stressful in other ways. We all need time to rest and process that before looking to the future. What lessons have we learned about what care options we should never lose again, and what might we want to keep as part of our lactation support work?

Chapter 7

Why we carry on

'Despite the stress, the hours, the exhaustion and the constant pushing a bus up a hill struggle, I will *never* do anything else now. Infant Feeding is my life, and I'm at peace with that.'
(HCP, Peer supporter)

If you're reading this book, nodding your head and thinking 'it's not just me, it really is a mess' then I wouldn't blame you. It is a mess. The profession is underfunded, undervalued and undermined. What is clear from the responses to the challenges of the role that despite this, the work is worth doing. More than worth doing. But why? Quite simply – families. Chapter four showed us that difficult relationships can occur between colleagues and many feel undervalued by the broader system; however, almost all respondents felt that the families who they worked with valued them. Look at this almost universal agreement to a series of statements in the survey exploring this:

- I feel valued by the families I support: 98.5%
- I usually feel like I'm doing a good job: 96.3%
- I feel privileged to be in my role: 98.5%
- I see a clear future in breastfeeding support: 81.7%

This brings me back to thinking about women's breastfeeding experiences more broadly. One thing that women often tell me in my research is that even though they are having all sorts of breastfeeding issues, they carry on because it's important to them for so many reasons. Breastfeeding doesn't need to be easy and stress free for them to continue, or indeed to even enjoy it. It is important in its own right. In fact, one of the best breastfeeding support posters I have seen was designed by Dorset NHS

Trust in the UK with the simple slogan 'We're not saying it's easy, we're saying it's worth it'. I bet you see the same day in, day out with many who you support.

Clearly any job has its challenges, especially if you are working with families at a vulnerable point in their lives. Many people often feel like throwing in the towel, but they don't. And a key question is why not? The answer to that is complex. In the survey participants were asked 'what keeps you going?' and there were numerous responses. I hope that you find your 'why' along with validation and reassurance in your role within these.

1. An intense need to support breastfeeding and good information

'Seeing happy healthy breastfeeding mothers and babies motivates me to carry on.' (IBCLC)

The ultimate reason for 'keeping on keeping on' in the survey was the simple fact that professionals and volunteers knew that they were making a difference. Supporting breastfeeding was at the heart of what drove individuals to continue, and they could see from their everyday encounters that their efforts were working. As one peer supporter in the UK simply said in relation to why she carried on – *'Because it helps mums to continue breastfeeding'*. Fundamentally this was such an important thing for many in the survey. Many simply felt an overwhelming need to support breastfeeding and that was what drove them to continue.

> *'I am driven by my passion for human milk as the biological norm of feeding a baby, supporting families reaching their feeding goals, nourishing the bond between baby and breastfeeding/chestfeeding parent and the health aspects of breast-/chestfeeding/human milk to feeding as a public health issue.' (IBCLC)*

A core part of this motivation was working to build a society that would be more supportive of breastfeeding. Respondents were very much motivated by the families in front of them, but by also knowing that with each family they helped it was one step closer to building an environment that truly supported breastfeeding and responsive parenting due to the ripple effect of having more positive breastfeeding experiences out there.

> *'Seeing the difference made to individuals by good breastfeeding support, and the wider cultural change in favour of breastfeeding that I believe we are starting to see motivates me to carry on. I can see the difference in families experiences and that's really important.' (Peer supporter)*

Another aspect to this was a common need to support the broader mission through ensuring that accurate and useful information circulated within communities and online.

> *'A great quote "be the change you want to see in the world" I want to dispel myths, and outdated advice, and listen to and support mums' choices.' (Peer supporter)*

Finally, some respondents experienced intense satisfaction from making a change within areas that did not believe in breastfeeding or the work that was being done. A dogged determination was present in many with a refusal to bow down to those who appeared to have an alternate mission of undermining breastfeeding and women's choices.

> *'I have to say I cherish the wins. There is so much against us but when we get a policy changed or come out triumphant against an article that has been derogatory about breastfeeding it does spur me on. I like winning even though it feels like we don't win very often. But while there is bad information out there I refuse to give up.' (IBCLC)*

Overall, we are back to that seemingly never-ending circle of the need for support driving your desire to give that support. Is this the ultimate 'chicken or egg' situation? Which came first? The need of so many families, or your desire to make a difference to them?

2. The satisfaction and reward of being able to help

'Nothing will ever be better than the feeling you get when you fix someone's pain or help them feel less anxious.' (Peer supporter)

Closely tied to the previous point was the immense personal reward when individuals were able to help others. This takes us back to the findings right at the start of this book where even though pressures related to the job role were stressful for many respondents, working with families on the ground was not. The feelings of reward, pride and satisfaction from helping a new mother or family continued to make the role worthwhile.

Many respondents were spurred on by the individual families that they supported reaching out to thank them. A day could be filled with tensions, barriers and paperwork and then a thank you card, or email would arrive and reignite a passion to continue.

> *'The notes of thanks, the words of appreciation, bumping into families I've helped (months or years later) and hearing their story about how things changed for the better after they saw me.' (IBCLC)*

This aspect of feeling valued has been shown to be protective against burnout and spurs professionals to stay in their role in midwifery[1] and nursing.[2] It appears that this aspect of the role may provide enough reward to outweigh the negative aspects. Indeed, in research exploring job satisfaction in healthcare professionals, direct contact with clients is often listed as one of the primary factors that leads to good job satisfaction, alongside elements such as supportive colleagues and opportunities for autonomy and independence.[3]

Additionally, research has shown that job satisfaction can help to reduce feelings of stress and burnout[4] and has been linked to better perceptions of care amongst patients.[5] All in all, a good relationship with those you are supporting is tightly entwined within good working relationships and wellbeing, even when there are broader negative aspects to the work.

3. The thought of what would happen without breastfeeding support

'If I don't do it then who will? I can so I should, I have a responsibility.' (Breastfeeding counsellor)

Many survey respondents were intensely aware that lactation support relied on passionate and motivated individuals continuing to work with families despite broader pressures of the role. Many carried the stark thought with them of what would happen if no one showed up. This was exacerbated by knowing that the system was heavily propped up on volunteers. If they didn't show up, who would?

> *'The thought of women not getting the support they need. Knowing the difference that one conversation can have for that mum and her baby.' (Breastfeeding counsellor)*

This realisation was a strong motivator to persevere and helped volunteers in particular to feel that what they were doing really made a difference, even if it felt like the system did not value them due to a lack of pay. However, as we have seen it can also cause an intense pressure to keep on giving when you really need a break. We will discuss the importance of also remembering to care for yourself later in chapter eight.

4. A duty to serve those in far tougher situations

Another motivator that came out strongly in survey responses was a calling to support and serve families that were in very challenging circumstances. Linked to the previous point of services relying on goodwill and volunteers, this aspect really focussed on families who had experienced significant traumas or stressors in their lives. Although we know that breastfeeding journeys can have long lasting implications for any family, these examples focussed on those for whom breastfeeding may be the last thread holding them together.

> *'I see families battling to feed their baby or child through terrible circumstances. In my role I have supported families where a child has cancer, or a likely incurable disease and mothers are fighting to ensure that their baby is breastfed or receives breast milk. Those families go through so much and need people like me to support them. How in all good faith could I turn round and tell them that I was giving up because it was too tough?' (Paediatric nurse)*

> *'In my practice I have served women for whom breastfeeding is an integral part of their recovery including those who have experienced sexual abuse and violence. Simply, I could never give up on them. It would destroy them to be failed by me too.' (IBCLC)*

Again, this comes back to 'wanting to make a difference' being a core motivation of the role. Being able to support those in the most challenging contexts feels deeply worthwhile and places many of the day-to-day stressors in context. Yes, a colleague was dismissive this morning and there's another media article denouncing breastfeeding, but here, on this ward, is where it really matters, and your energy can be directed to make a real difference. The challenging and sometimes tragic circumstances of those you support help to put it all in perspective.

5. A desire to 'give back' to the system

As discussed in chapter three, it is often our own challenging experiences that draw us into a role working or volunteering in lactation support. Many survey participants talked about how they had a strong desire to give back to the system and make a difference in the way that someone else made a difference to them. They understood how it felt to struggle and the difference that good support made. They also knew that no matter how challenging the role could be, there would always be families to whom you could make a real difference. That is what motivated them to keep getting up each morning and trying to support others over and over again.

> 'Everyday I remember how I felt when someone reached out to me. I am doing this in return for the support I received and if I can make a small difference in how someone feels about themselves and their baby it's worth it. Kind of hoping to repeat the feeling I got for someone else.' (Peer supporter)

Reciprocity - or the feeling of giving back - is a known motivator for volunteers across different settings. It stems from wanting others to have the same support that you did, feeling a debt of gratitude and simply wanting to play your part in a cycle of community support. Feelings of solidarity and connection with others who are going through the same thing are also common, with some volunteers finding that helping others helps to further heal their own pain and memories.[6] Indeed, in recent research that I conducted with Dr Natalie Shenker, a key motivator of going on to donate human milk was having received it for your own baby and wanting to pay back to the system and the community that supported you.[7]

6. Feeling part of a supportive community of practice

Related to discussion in chapter four which considered the stress of disconnection, another aspect that motivated supporters to continue was feeling like they were part of a team or community of those working to support lactation. The support of colleagues and confidants spurred supporters to continue. Those in this situation felt valued and connected to those working alongside them and were proud of being part of a team of supporters.

> 'I carry on because of my peers. I see their strength and determination in battling tough challenges with grace. They inspire me and make me proud to consider them friends. I am in awe of what they achieve. Without them I would feel lonely but they pick me up and carry me when I need it and me them. I owe it to them to continue.' (IBCLC)

> 'I'd be lost without the other girls. They understand me and support me and I would hate not to be part of this team. Obviously we are here to support families but the friendships that have developed through my peer supporting reach far beyond what we do on a Thursday morning. We know each other's babies, partners and family members. We are family and I'd never want to lose that.' (Peer supporter)

This 'one person' or group of like-minded colleagues often appeared to be enough to outweigh negativity, misunderstanding and criticism from other professionals who were not supportive of infant feeding roles. It is reflective of the broader literature around how childhood resilience develops and the concept that when children are living in adverse circumstances having one positive attachment relationship can sometimes be enough to partly outweigh absent or harmful relationships.[8] This one supportive and nurturing individual who encourages and supports a child's emotional needs can help them build positive self-belief and resilience against stressors. It feels as if the same is true within the lactation profession. As long as you have that one person or group of peers who genuinely support and understand you, then you can face the world for another day.

Research with other healthcare professional groups has clearly shown the importance of good working relationships with colleagues in helping foster resilience and reduce stress.[9] In an aptly titled book chapter focussing on midwifery entitled *'Relationships- the glue that holds it all together'*, five midwifery leaders hone in on the value of connections between midwives for overcoming the stressors and challenges of the role.[10] These positive working relationships have long been identified as a crucial element of preventing burnout especially in times of challenge and adversity.[11]

Within this concept, the positive working relationships that many professionals and volunteers have with families is fundamental. This isn't just about helping families to thrive and have better infant feeding outcomes, but also about the relationship that develops between you and families over time. Sometimes this is more fleeting but occasionally it can last a lifetime.

'I can be having a terrible day and then I bump into someone I supported 20, even 30 years ago and their baby is a grown up but they still remember what I said. What is there better than that to keep you going?' (Breastfeeding counsellor)

Research has shown just how protective these connections with others can be in terms of reducing feelings of stress but also keeping us connected to a field. In one study with midwives, relationships with colleagues and parents were felt to be some of the most rewarding aspects of the role.[10] There is a suggestion that these relationships can be an important buffer against stress. For example, having 'like minded peers' with whom to offload and share the challenges arose in another midwifery study in New Zealand exploring resilience.[1] These relationships with colleagues and families are often felt to outweigh the stressors of healthcare professional roles[11] particularly if management relationships are also strong.[12]

7. Professional pride and identity

Finally, many respondents carried a strong sense of professional pride and identity in their work. Over and above the role of supporting families, many were proud to be connected to the lactation world and felt that it was an important and valuable role.

> 'It is the nearest thing to a 'career' I have been able to have and I think I am good at it. I work with aspiring Breastfeeding counsellors whose enthusiasm and idealism is infectious. I feel valued by my organisation and they are flexible.' (Breastfeeding counsellor)

> 'I love, love, love being able to call myself an IBCLC and being able to call this group of professionals from around the world my colleagues.' (IBCLC)

In one study exploring resilience amongst midwives, having a strong sense of identity and having a love for midwifery practice were identified as core factors in the development of resilience against role stressors and a desire to continue in the field.[13] In a similar study in New Zealand this concept arose again with many finding 'joy' in their role and holding real pride in being part of the profession.[1] This pride, sense of identity and sheer connection to the role and what it means is indeed evident across a number of studies in midwifery and nursing.[14,15] It really does represent that concept of a 'calling' to the profession, or a strong vocational passion that is often sustained no matter what the role throws in your face.

Others felt that it was simply what they were 'good' or skilled at. They found the role intuitive and easy, despite the challenges they were presented with and felt that they had found their fit in life. It helped them feel like a competent individual and gave them a purpose. For some this was the first time they had 'achieved' in a role or gained a qualification and that filled them with pride.

> *'I dropped out of school at 16 and was never considered to be the clever one at home. I never thought I would be one to have an internationally recognised qualification and get to show parents my certificates. It's really changed the way I feel about myself and what I'm good at and capable of.'* (IBCLC)

Unfortunately for some this meant that they were not paid for their work, fitting in with many of those memes on social media that draw a Venn diagram but with no overlap for 'things I am good at' and 'things that pay my bills'. Despite this, the draw to the role and feelings of fulfilment and personal success were so strong that they fitted this around a full time job or even reduced hours at work in order to be able to do it.

> *'Pay would be nice I'm sure but the role offers me so much more than money could ever bring.'* (Peer supporter)

> *'I wish I was paid for what I do but I'll never give it up. It's like a drug to me – it's addictive at making me feel good in a way nothing else does!'* (Peer supporter)

Take home message: There are so many positives to be had working in this role and this is something that should never be lost amongst any conflict, misunderstanding or paperwork. Hold onto that pride, connection and feelings of gratitude that families offer. Haters gonna hate and all that. Or remember the words of one peer supporter who simply said *'What we do matters'*.

Chapter 8

Tools for support

'You need to invest in you, your mental health matters too. You can't pour water from an empty cup, so take the time to fill yourself back up.' (Peer supporter)

In this penultimate chapter I wanted to focus on some strategies for supporting you. I have brought together ideas from participants in the survey in relation to what helps them to cope with the pressures of a lactation support role, alongside broader evidence around mental health and stress, drawing on research exploring what works in supporting other health care professionals. I know that in stressful situations it is all too easy to fall back on crutches that are not helpful in the long term. For example, in research with midwives who were working with women in stressful circumstances, many talked about the unhealthy coping strategies they used. This included 'taking the stress home' and getting involved with arguments with their partner or shouting at their children. Others felt emotionally disengaged or distracted at home. Others turned to too much alcohol.[1]

Whilst I won't rule out the medicinal properties of the occasional *'sitting in a hot tub with a gin'* (see forthcoming suggestion from one peer supporter), I do know that there are many more useful ways to also support your wellbeing. There are a wide range of ideas here and I'm certainly not offering a panacea nor expecting that everything will work for everyone all of the time. Some may appeal to you, while some may make you recoil. Some may feel impossible to you due to a lack of time, money or physical limitations. I do hope there is something that you can draw strength from – and let me know on social media if you have any other ideas that work well for you! If you'd like to explore this topic in more depth I would really recommend the book

'Nurturing Maternity Staff' by Dr Jan Smith. Although the book is focussed on those working across maternity care, there is a lot of overlap of stressors and challenges between the roles, and Jan has some great therapy techniques in terms of supporting your wellbeing.

1. Focus on building supportive relationships

'Develop good working relationships with other breastfeeding supporters and health care professionals - we are stronger together.' (Breastfeeding counsellor)

Focussing on building a support circle around you can be vital in what can feel like a really lonely role at times. If you're not lucky enough to have a supportive team of allies around you already, we really recommend reaching out and building your own if possible. This could be through joining supportive social media groups designed specifically for lactation professionals or supporters. Some recommended ones include:

- Specific organisational groups for members such as the Association of Breastfeeding Mothers Trained and Training for those associated with the charity
- Lactogenesis II
- UK IBCLCs in Private Practice
- UNICEF UK BFI
- Hospital Infant Feeding Network
- Breastfeeding for Doctors

It is also worth forming your own smaller group of friends and allies to offload in a safe and private space, in person or via online messaging. Just anywhere where you can rant and people will understand – or as one IBCLC described *'Somewhere you can share, relax, cry, work together to change things, feel supported and help each other'*. Never underestimate the restorative aspects of being heard and understood by like-minded peers.

A core part of this circle of allies is the mutual support element. Remember to check in with others you work alongside (literally or more metaphorically within the online world), asking how your colleagues are doing. Not only is this mutually respectful but talking to others about the stressors they face can help reduce your own anxiety and intrusive thoughts about not being 'good enough'. I'm betting they have similar challenging thoughts or pressures of their own, and sometimes simply knowing that others find this difficult at times can really help. It can also help to hold each other accountable to things like taking a break, caring for ourselves and striving for some semblance of work-life balance (more on this part in a bit).

It's also important to consider here for a moment who we might have potentially overlooked and, through no fault on either side, not included in our support and mentoring networks. We will return to this point at the end of the chapter, but when we think about who is benefitting from informal networks of support, is anyone missing? Friendship, connection and emotional support are 'unseen' ways in which we grow, develop or sustain ourselves in any role. They are a way of passing on knowledge, wisdom and skill and fostering resilience.

Related to looking to others for support is having someone who you can talk to in a more formalised way. Several survey respondents brought up the importance of good quality, regular supervision. This we know can play a vital part in helping us process and offload our concerns and emotions related to families and scenarios that we have been supporting.

'Good quality supervision and debrief is really important - indeed, I'd suggest we're dangerous without it. I take Supervision and use reflective practice, reflective writing and debriefing seriously as a vital part of my work. I am a supervisor for my breastfeeding counsellor colleagues and think supervision and reflection should be mandatory for those of us working in support roles.' (IBCLC)

It's also a really good idea to try and spend some time focussing on positive breastfeeding experiences and those you *have* been able to help. This is such an important thing to remember. Often we focus on the challenging situations we face in infant feeding and forget that actually, many families out there are having a happy and successful breastfeeding journey. A version of gratitude thinking may work here where at the end of the day you list three things that were positive in the world of infant feeding (some days treating this more loosely than others…!).

'We should do things that make us feel that our work is valuable. For example, seeing more mothers successfully and happily breastfeeding their baby.' (Breastfeeding counsellor)

'Remember to count the positives too and don't let them get overshadowed by the setbacks. They are there, you just may need to look harder for them some days.' (IBCLC)

Finally, do remember to connect with those outside of the breastfeeding world. As one IBCLC noted *'I spend time with people who are NOT involved in breastfeeding talking about other subjects so that I can 'switch off' for a while.'* It's great to take a step back and remind yourself that other things are going on in the world and spend some time talking to people who are never going to bring up faltering growth or debate the best way to treat mastitis!

2.   Try to develop and stick to boundaries

'I am an all or nothing person (I highly suspect I have ADHD with breastfeeding as my area of hyper focus) I would always guide others to make time for themselves, deactivate their social media or mute notifications if it was getting too much for them and assuring them that taking a step back for the time they need wouldn't stop them being able to give support in the future if they felt that way.' (Peer supporter)

I lost track of the number of times in the survey that participants stated the importance of developing boundaries to protect and prioritise your wellbeing. As one survey respondent emphasised:

'Boundaries are extremely important. It's vital to me that I have a life outside of breastfeeding and live it!' (IBCLC)

This is so tough to uphold because of all the reasons discussed in the book. You care about the families you support. You care about doing a good job. You care about making a difference. And then you worry about what's happening when you're not there. It's so easy to feel like you're not doing enough or must always be available.

But it's at times like these that we need to afford ourselves the same kindness as we do the families we support. How often do we tell a new mother that it's ok that she needs a break? That she's not selfish for needing time alone? That she should prioritise self-care and her own needs? Treat yourself like you would treat that new family you were caring for. As another one participant in the survey described:

'When I am with a parent (in-person, phone, online, etc.), I am totally with that parent, but when I leave, I let it go. I don't own another's breastfeeding issue - I'll do what I can to help - but I don't carry another's issue home.' (IBCLC).

There is no one 'correct' working pattern or number of hours that you should be working on relaxing (bar sensible recommendations around sleep and self-care). You will need to work out how you function best and how that fits in with other roles and relationships. You might be thriving, happy and totally fine working 60 hours a week. Conversely you might be struggling with 15 hours. We're not all starting from the same energy and availability baseline - nor indeed an inclination one!

Some specific tips for boundary settings suggested by participants included:

- Having a separate work phone and personal phone – and turn off your work phone at the end of your day.

- Separating personal and work social media – likewise just have work social media on your work phone so you do not see notifications when you switch it off

- Formalising working hours and trying to stick to those where possible.

- Turn off social media notifications or use an app on your phone that locks you out during set periods.

- Scheduling leisure activities in your diary and treating them with the importance of work commitments.

- Having a reflective diary that you complete at the end of each day and then shut and put away somewhere you can't see it.

- Developing an end of working day ritual - almost akin to a bedtime routine you might share with a parent of a young baby. The same principles apply!

- Leaving your laptop at home if you go away / phone downstairs at night.

Another big one identified in the survey was learning to say no. Oh this sounds so simple, doesn't it? Just say no! It's incredibly hard to do because of all the reasons given above, but if you start small you will see that typically nothing bad happens. After far too many years of saying yes to everything I started an 'I said no' list where I note down everything that I say no to and the time it would have taken up. You can see how much it adds up.

Also, when someone asks you to do something, ask yourself what you would have to give up to do it, as I'm pretty sure you're already fairly busy. It's easy to imagine a hypothetical time in the future when you'll have time for this new thing, but will you really? If you do it, will it mean you can't do another part of your role? Or will it take away from time with family? Or your hobbies, or downtime? Is it worth it? This technique allows you more time to prioritise what you really value - and makes it less likely that you'll be angry at your past self for saying yes!

It can help to involve others in your boundary setting. Making plans with family and friends means you are less likely to back out. And by this we don't just mean spending more time caring for children or others, but rather engaging with others in a way that nurtures you. If you are an introvert, make plans with yourself to read a book or watch a film and hold yourself as accountable to yourself as if you were your friend.

Several participants in the survey also talked about finding strength in their faith, because the teachings of their faith encouraged rest or other activities. I'm not suggesting you go and join a religious group simply to get a break, but there is certainly something to take away from such messages even if you do not follow a religion. Breaks are important and sacred because they help you to rest and recover and continue to serve in your work.

'Have a weekly "Sabbath"! Every Friday night, we shut down everything related to work/ income/ producing, and focus on family and our faith community.' (IBCLC)

'I go to church twice each Sunday and often spend the afternoon with our group. It is non-negotiable. It's part of a wider promise to God and my church community but it does also mean I have a routine and switch off.' (Nurse).

If you are really struggling with this, it could help to consider working with a life coach or counsellor to try and work out why. Is it just that you really enjoy working so many hours? Or is it a tendency for perfectionism at play, or the habit of distracting yourself from other issues by keeping yourself overworked? Why don't you value your own time and space? Who taught you that?

3. Prioritise activities that you enjoy and calm your system

'Self care first because we can't pour from an empty cup.'
(Breastfeeding counsellor)

Once you've put those boundaries in place to give you that time to focus on you then taking time to calm your frazzled and overworked system is important. It's about putting yourself first, giving yourself time and space to decompress and the physiological benefits that different activities can bring.

Four core ideas that participants in the survey discussed were a) being creative b) being active c) getting outside d) physical touch. At this point I want to put in a huge disclaimer that we realise that workloads, family life, financial strains and limitations of our body can all make these tricky. However, finding something that works for you is so worth it, even if it seems like an impossibility. Keep reminding yourself that in all of this you matter too.

Harnessing your creativity

Research documenting the mental health benefits of spending time being creative is mounting. Being creative in whatever way appeals to you and fits with your lifestyle has shown to be restorative across a whole range of mental health aspects from simply needing some time to focus on your wellbeing through to more serious challenges.[2] There are several reasons for this. Often keeping your hands physically busy and thinking about where to put that next stitch or colour or word in your poem helps soothe and calm your brain. It can be distracting from unwanted and intrusive thoughts. There's also a lovely sense of accomplishment of producing something and a sense of achievement from successfully finishing a 'job' (in contrast to the never-ending flood of parents needing support). The rhythmic nature of many crafts can help soothe a frazzled brain and system. You can feel your shoulders relax.

You might choose to do something completely unrelated to your work such as knitting a blanket or completing a jigsaw. Other people prefer to do something therapeutic such as writing angry or hard-hitting poems or blogs to get the frustration out of their head and connect with and resonate with others. Some find comfort in work related crafts such as knitting breasts or tiny baby clothes. Basically, it is about whatever works for you.

If you're stuck for ideas, activities mentioned in the survey including knitting, crochet, paint by numbers, free painting, drawing, colouring books, jigsaws, calligraphy, felting, paper cutting, making clothes, woodwork, home decorating, writing, poetry, and even website design. Inspiration can also be found in the 'Maternal journal' by Laura Godfrey-Isaacs and Samantha McGowan. Although primarily aimed at pregnant and new parents I absolutely adore the artwork and different creative ideas in this book and would fully recommend it for anyone wanting to stimulate their creativity.

Another option that works for some is to sign up to do some further study related to your role. I know this might seem counterintuitive (As one Breastfeeding counsellor declared 'I started a Masters, I wouldn't necessarily recommend that!'), but it seems an increasingly common decision, especially amongst those who are more established and settled in their lactation role or whose children are a little older now (or in other words amongst those who have hit, or are about to hit their 40s or 50s).

It helps because it provides another focus and feels like you are moving forward and opening up your future options. It can also feel like you are doing something positive to support the families you work with. And let's face it, it can also serve as a distraction from everything else that is going on!

Getting active

Another helpful strategy to tackle stress is to spend time doing something more physical, if you are able. We know that exercise helps reduce physical symptoms of stress, improve mental health and can help reduce inflammation in the body. When we are stressed our bodies react by raising our stress hormones and consequently our heart rate and blood pressure. This response was designed as a protective mechanism to help us escape from whatever was stressing us (i.e. trying to attack, threaten or eat us). However, in our modern-day world where running away from or fighting stress is more difficult, this response becomes problematic. Stress increases inflammation in the body which is in turn associated with many negative health outcomes. Exercise can help reduce that.[3]

I'm not suggesting you take up ultra-running (ok, I might try to convince you, but feel free to nod and ignore me) but trying to take time to fit in more exercise, or an activity that works for you, into your life really can be worth it. It can feel impossible or almost indulgent at times, but your body will thank you for it, if only because it will get a chance to unfurl after a long day at your laptop. Anything that raises your heart rate can work well including stomping across a moor or through woodland, practising yoga at home or swimming. Weightlifting is also important for female longer-term health, especially once you hit menopause. I also recommend the therapeutic practice of hitting a punch bag.

If you have an illness or a disability that makes this difficult, there are increasingly more classes that are more inclusive such as seated yoga and tai chi. An upside of pandemic lockdowns was the increase in accessible online classes. Whatever options you follow, the core focus is on feeling stronger, calmer and more able to take on the day.

Ring-fenced time to be active or exercise can help sort out all the thoughts in your head while your body is active. Sometimes people in caring professions (and women more broadly) struggle to take time to prioritise themselves especially if they have small children. I understand all the barriers and I have very much been there myself. Yet the headspace that a walk in the woods can bring is so beneficial that I think it should be viewed as an essential 'work task'.

Remember, if you can put it in your diary and treat it like any other health appointment (ok, we know you can end up skipping those too... but you get the gist... and also, don't skip it!). Others suggested an active commute if walking or cycling is possible in your role (or keeping trainers in your locker and running home once a week). This is easier if you live locally rather than 30 miles away obviously... unless you really do like ultra-running!

Get outside

Spending time in nature (known as 'greenspace') came up so many times in the survey, whether that was a walk with the kids, sitting with a coffee watching the sea with a friend or simply taking in the view at the top of a hill. As one midwife shared *'Take the time to stop and stare'*.

Gardening also featured heavily, alone or with others. As did the increasingly common mid-life survival activity choice for women of cold water swimming (known apparently as 'blue space'). Time in nature has been shown to help reduce stress and improve mental health both amongst those who are generally feeling frazzled and those with mental health issues. As one breastfeeding counsellor said, *'I walk the dog - fresh air and exercise give me an opportunity to think and put everything into perspective'*.

Alongside physiological stress reduction, reasons proposed for this positive impact include the feeling of escape/getting away from it all, having time and space to reflect, distraction from worrying thoughts, having structure and plans, learning new skills / feeling good at something, and simply enjoying the activity.[4] There are a surprising number of research papers published on the mental health benefits of allotments and horticultural therapy.[5] And fortunately or unfortunately depending on your thoughts about temperature and early mornings, there is a growing body of research highlighting the benefits of cold water swimming. It increases all the feel-good hormones (dopamine, serotonin and endorphins), boosts your white blood cell count and reduces stress hormones.[6] Personally, I still remain unconvinced!

Harness the power of physical touch and bodywork

Finally, physical treatments such as massage, spa days, meditation and other bodywork were often mentioned. We know that massage and other therapies can have a healing effect on the body, helping to reduce physical signs of stress and even improve mental health.[7] However, I absolutely realise that if you're frazzled, juggling three young children, or worried about money (or just dislike strangers touching you), then you might laugh out loud at these suggestions! Saying that, don't underestimate the calming benefits of some time spent meditating or focussing on your breathing. Self-massage can also help to invoke some of the calming response with research suggesting it can also help reduce blood pressure, lower stress hormones and reduce symptoms of depression.[8]

Meditation[9] and mindfulness[10] exercises can also have similar impacts. Indeed, meditation was recommended by one peer supporter in the survey who practised this before and after meeting with parents. If you are feeling frazzled, doubting yourself or having 'stage fright' it can really help to calm and ground you before you step into the work zone. One breathing exercise that can help is a yoga breathing exercise known as alternate nostril breathing. To do this you use your thumb to close one nostril and breathe slowly and steadily out of the other one. Then switch. And repeat a few times. Keeping your eyes closed can help. Essentially the exercise focuses on steadying your breathing and calming your system.

Grounding is another great exercise if you feel yourself stressed and panicking. Sit quietly and notice the things around you. Pick either a colour or a sense (i.e. smell) and name what is going on in your environment. You might choose five things that you can see that are green. Five things you can smell. Five sounds you can hear. This helps calm your system and bring you back to the moment.

Some final ideas

Of course, not everything that you do has to be evidence based and 'worthy'. The key element here is taking time for you, doing something that you want to do, with no one making demands on your time. Some of our favourite suggestions from the survey include:

'Take some time out to do something you enjoy, I take myself to bed with a good book.' (Peer supporter)

'I crochet - stabbing yarn and swearing a bit helps...!' (Peer supporter)

'Any activity outside breastfeeding area: gardening, travelling...reading (not breastfeeding literature!).' (IBCLC)

'I garden and help keep bees - very separate to breastfeeding work and volunteering.' (HCP, Breastfeeding counsellor)

'Read fiction, walk... mostly seek comfort in kindred spirits.' (HCP, Peer supporter)

'I bake! Get my kids involved in it or days out. Laughing lots, taking yoga classes, having fun.' (Peer supporter)

'Exercise. Time with friends. Finding a good babysitter!' (Breastfeeding counsellor)

'Hot tub in my garden helps me chills out, we all need an hour with a gin in the tub and we'll all be calmer.' (Peer supporter)

4. Be kinder to yourself

'Be sure to treat yourself with as much care as you give to your clients.' (Peer supporter)

If we think back to the earlier chapter on the challenges of empathy, perfectionism and impostor syndrome being combined with a deep passion for lactation work, then one core suggestion is to make sure that you are treating yourself with the kindness and forgiveness that you would a close friend. The importance of this was central throughout survey responses showing how common the tendency is to beat ourselves up and the wisdom gained by others who have managed to overcome this.

It is so common to worry that we should have done something differently or offered alternative guidance. We dwell on our words wondering if we accidentally did harm. We worry about families long after we leave their home. We ruminate over those who might have been harmed by our factual messages because they've had such difficult feeding experiences in the past. We worry about our reputations and how we are coming across.

Tell yourself just how brilliant you are. It might sound cheesy, but you could ask a trusted friend or colleague to list the positive qualities they see in you (with you repaying the favour should they wish). If you don't feel comfortable doing this, try to step outside yourself a little and imagine you are talking to yourself as a kind friend. What do they see in you? We keep repeating this but treat yourself with the kindness you would treat a good friend. Would you judge them if they messed up or weren't 100% on the ball all the time? No? Well don't do it to yourself.

Another trick here is to apply the kindness and wisdom we share with parents about caring for their baby. So much of what we urge parents to think about is actually just as true for us too, even down to the phrase that often divides the lactation world 'never give up on a bad day'. On a serious note, we tell parents to be kind to themselves, that everyone is learning and that it's ok to feel like you don't know what you're doing. We remind them to take a break and look after themselves as they can't pour from an empty cup (and that they matter too). Why don't we apply that same kindness to ourselves?

Here are the top tips from those who have been there and understand some of what you are feeling:

'Remind yourself that even if you are only able to give a family an informed choice, then you have done your job regardless of the decisions they make.' (Peer supporter)

'Help those who want to be helped.' (Breastfeeding counsellor)

'Focus on those you help. Do not get into arguments with those who question you. Don't engage with those who don't value breastfeeding.' (Breastfeeding counsellor)

'Don't take other peoples choices personally. Our role is to validate, inform, and then support mothers in THEIR CHOICES. When we respect women's choices it's easier to let go of the one's we don't agree with.' (Peer supporter)

'I've been lucky to have had mentoring, I know the difference between "responsible for" and "responsible to" and I remind myself I am not solely responsible for every mother or parent.' (Breastfeeding counsellor)

'Realise that we can only do so much and we aren't responsible for all of infant feeding. If we make a difference to one mum then we're winning.' (Peer supporter)

'Help the mum in front of you the best you can, you can not control their circumstance or change the wider cultural context for that mum. Don't over think it and stay away from the trolls!!!!' (Breastfeeding counsellor)

5. Challenge those feelings of impostor syndrome and perfectionism

Sometimes it's the role that stresses us out, but occasionally the way we personally react to stress can make things feel more challenging. Sometimes a role may feel even more stressful because of our own high standards or negative self-talk. Clearly, working on any feelings of impostor syndrome or perfectionism are not going to magically make everything better if you're surrounded by families who are in deeply stressful situations. However, if you're finding yourself doubting yourself or putting too much pressure on yourself to support all the families, then reflecting on what drives you to act this way may help relieve some of this stress.

It's normal to carry doubts, especially in the face of so many challenges whilst supporting families against the system. Doubts are normal and healthy and keep us grounded. In fact, we'd be a bit worried if you never *ever* doubted yourself as it would probably mean you have become numb, disconnected or overly confident. Having the occasional doubt or reflection is one thing when compared to regular anxiety and beating yourself up over your every decision.

Overcoming feelings of impostor syndrome and perfectionism is a three-pronged approach. The first thing that can help can be to remind yourself that doubts and mistakes are normal. The second is to reflect on what you have achieved. Finally, the third is to experiment with imperfection. Some tips for overcoming these issues are:

- Remind yourself that everyone (or the sensible ones) doubts themselves at some point and that imperfection and mistakes are common and normal. If you're not convinced, ask a more experienced colleague or peer that you trust whether they've ever made a mistake. I bet they'll laugh and reel off a list of daft-in-hindsight stories.

- Recognise what you do know. Make a list of your qualifications and experience. Add in achievements no matter how big or small. Collate feedback from families. Keep emails and correspondence in a file on your desktop or phone. Read your list. Re-read your list. Aren't you great?

- Try to slowly wean yourself off your need to be perfect. You are the one most likely driving your expectations rather than anyone else. What would happen if you reduced the pressure you put on yourself? Would your progress irreparably slow down? Would your reputation disappear? We bet not, but you need to take the first step in tentatively experimenting with your comfort point. Make a list of all the things you are putting pressure on yourself to do. What can go? Do you really need to see that family with the non-urgent issue immediately? Try saying no when people ask you to do things. Start small. How does it feel? What could you do with the saved time?

- Alternatively try lowering your standards very slightly. Obviously, this is contextual and if you are dealing with an important feeding issue, don't drop your standards! Can other tasks be reduced? If you're running a social media site, can you save time by not faffing over it being perfect? Write it, check it over, get it out there. What happens? Is the world still turning?

- An important reflection is to think about what is causing you to feel this way? Where did these feelings of doubt or a need to be perfect come from? Why are you feeling so much pressure or doubt? What are you afraid of and why? Who told you that you weren't good enough or were only good enough if you were overachieving? Understanding why you feel this way helps you stop and think about how you could move forward. You might be able to do this alone, or you might benefit from some coaching or counselling to get to the root of the issue.

6. Choose whose voice you listen to

This is particularly true for those of us on social media but extends across the lactation world (well, across any workplace or field really). There will always be people who criticise you whether that's a colleague or peer, a family you tried to help or a stranger on social media. Sometimes this criticism is constructive and valid and designed to help you grow and improve your skills. We would try to frame this as feedback rather than criticism. At other times it's the absolute opposite and designed to undermine you, either because the individual is a bully, vindictive or simply jealous. Distinguishing between these intentions and deciding whose voice you listen to is a critical part of staying sane.

It's at this point that I always revert to talking about the queen of dealing with critics – Professor Brené Brown. If you haven't read her books on belonging, shame and connection then I really recommend them as they are full of strategies to reflect and act on criticism. One of my favourites is from her book Daring Greatly where Brené talks about how she carries a small piece of paper in her wallet with the names of people whose opinion actually matters to her.[11] If you're not on that list you're not getting into Brené's head.

Who would (and who should) be on your list? Your partner? Family? Children? Trusted colleagues and peers? Absolutely. Who shouldn't? That peer who you know holds a grudge because you got an opportunity that they did not. That stranger on the internet intent on trolling you. That colleague in work who shows narcissistic traits and is intent on bullying. In other words, if everything fell apart tomorrow, who would be there for you? It's *those* people who should be on that piece of paper.

Another brilliant piece is Brené's fantastic YouTube video 'Why Your Critics Don't Count'.[12] In this video she refers to a famous quote by Thomas Roosevelt:[13]

"It is not the critic who counts; not the man who points out how the strong man stumbles, or where the doer of deeds could have done them better. The credit belongs to the man who is actually in the arena, whose face is marred by dust and sweat and blood; who strives valiantly; who errs, who comes short again and again, because there is no effort without error and shortcoming; but who does actually strive to do the deeds; who knows great enthusiasms, the great devotions; who spends himself in a worthy cause; who at the best knows in the end the triumph of high achievement, and who at the worst, if he fails, at least fails while daring greatly, so that his place shall never be with those cold and timid souls who neither know victory nor defeat."

In relation to this Brené simply says, '*If you're not in the arena getting your ass kicked I'm not interested in your feedback*'. This says it all. Are the people who are criticising or bullying you reaching families with the same skills and kindness? Are they working with the same pressures? Have they put themselves out there in the same way? Most likely not – so why are you still listening? Don't be afraid to judiciously use the handy block or mute feature on social media.

Of course, if criticism has turned to flat out bullying there are steps you could and should take. The ACAS website has some great information on spotting signs of bullying and what action you can take.[14] Although there is no formal definition of bullying, in terms of what likely counts as bullying behaviour it includes aspects such as

- Spreading malicious rumours
- Frequent put downs especially in front of others
- Being given a heavier workload than others
- Humiliating, offensive or threatening posts on social media
- Undermining your authority

The website notes that bullying does not necessarily have to be 'downward' e.g. from someone in a senior role or with more experience. It can be 'upward' from those you are line managing or leading, including behaviours such as showing continued disrespect, refusing to complete tasks, spreading rumours and trying to deliberately make you look like you are not doing your job properly.

It is important to be aware of any bullying behaviour that could be considered harassment. This occurs when the bullying is occurring due to any of the protected characteristics under the Equality Act 2010 and includes bullying specific to age, disability, gender reassignment, race, religion or belief, sex or sexual orientation.

How you handle bullying depends on who is bullying you and where you are working. If you are in an organisation you can, and should, report bullying behaviour to your line manager or boss who has a duty of care to respond to you and the situation. You might wish to keep a diary of the bullying instances, or create a file of 'evidence' e.g. aggressive or discriminatory emails, social media posts or other occurrences. This can include behaviours that others do not witness, although obviously that is more problematic to prove, and we know many bullies are adept at erasing any evidence trail. If you are self-employed it is more challenging but it is possible to report people's bullying behaviour to their organisation or governing body.

Another thing that we can all do is to speak out when we see others being bullied. It supports professional behaviour, individuals and helps others to gain the confidence to call out bullies. As above you can also block, mute and report on social media. The Royal College of Obstetricians and Gynaecologists also have a very useful toolkit designed to address bullying in the workplace. You can learn more about spotting the signs of bullying and what to do if you have been bullied or witness bullying behaviour.[15]

7. Seek professional help if you need it

Finally, if you are really struggling with burnout, compassion fatigue or anxiety and depression all the 'be kind to yourself' and 'do some knitting' messages aren't really going to cut it. Knowing the difference between being frustrated and needing a break, and clinical signs of burnout and mental health issues is really important.

Danger signs

The NHS lists the following signs of stress and burnout. Some of these symptoms are normal reactions to stressful events that occur. They pass after the pressure eases, or you have had a chance to relax and focus on yourself for a bit. If these symptoms still do not ease, or your stress is unrelenting then this could be a sign that you would benefit from some professional support:

- Feeling overwhelmed
- Having racing thoughts or difficulty concentrating
- Feeling irritable
- Feeling constantly worried, anxious or scared
- Feeling a lack of self-confidence
- Trouble sleeping or feel tired all the time
- Avoiding things / people you have problems with
- Eating more or less than usual
- Drinking or smoking more than usual

There are tools online for considering whether you are experiencing dangerous levels of burnout including on the British Medical Association[17] and NHS websites.[16] Some of the common signs of anxiety and depression are often:

- Feeling tense, nervous or tearful
- Feeling angry or frustrated
- Low confidence and self esteem
- Being unable to relax and fearing the worst happening

- Worrying about the past or future
- Not being able to sleep or eat (or eating or sleeping more)
- Having difficulty concentrating
- Feeling on edge or lacking energy
- Intrusive traumatic memories or obsessive thoughts
- Not getting any enjoyment out of life or feeling hopeless
- Having suicidal thoughts or thoughts about harming yourself

If you spot these signs in yourself (or your colleagues and friends) please do reach out for support. There are some recommended sources of support at the end of the book, but a good starting place would be an occupational health department (if you have one), GP, local counsellor or charity support such as MIND in the UK. Don't let your brain tell you that it's not serious enough or you don't matter. No matter how you are feeling you deserve the support to feel calmer and stronger.

Take home message: I've said it before several times already, but I'll say it again - give yourself the same kindness, care and permission to look after yourself as you do the parents that you care for!

Chapter 9

A manifesto for change

Drawing this book to a close, a key question remains. We can take steps to care for our mental and physical health but what needs to change at a societal level so that supporting breastfeeding is a smoother journey in the future? When you read through the list below you will most likely note that there is a lot of similarity between what needs to change to better support new families and what needs to change to help those who are supporting them. We are all working and caring within the same bubble and affected by the broader structures that interfere with and damage breastfeeding.

What did those in the survey want to see changed? Three broad aspects emerged: changes to the way breastfeeding was viewed by government, healthcare organisations and society; changes to breastfeeding service delivery that would make a difference to families; and changes to the structure of breastfeeding support roles.

1. Government, healthcare organisation and societal support for breastfeeding

'A government and society that recognised the importance of breastfeeding from all perspectives: health; immunological; emotional; developmental; economic and environmental to name but a few!' (IBCLC)

The absolute number one recommendation for change was more funding. Investment was needed in the system to enable resources across the perinatal period.

> *'I would like to know that if I suggest a mother seek further health professional advice for anything she needs, that she will get it.' (Peer supporter)*

Others were more specific in what needed to be funded. Notably, although many did refer to increased funding to be able to support posts, it was often actually the smaller things that respondents felt would make all the difference. Venue hire was one of the most frequently suggested specific requests. Perhaps this is a small cost, but indeed when you have no budget to be able to provide a breastfeeding support group or clinic, then how do your trained staff and supporters reach families?

> *'Guaranteed funding for breastfeeding groups, access to funding for resources, paid breastfeeding support workers, higher volunteer numbers, meaningful government and NHS endorsement of breastfeeding.' (Peer supporter)*

The need for more investment is not earth-shattering news and indeed feels in part like a tired and repetitive conversation - but it is the one thing that is vitally important to continue pushing. Without secured investment in the long term, how do we plan? How do we move forward confident that our efforts won't be pulled from underneath us? How do we feel protected enough to relax into our roles and focus more energy on supporting mothers and families?

This highlights a major issue in breastfeeding promotion. All too often governments are ok at policy messaging but weak on following through with the tools needed to actually enable a supportive environment for breastfeeding to be created. Most governments around the world will have a statement that supports something along the lines of the World Health Organisation guidelines that babies should be exclusively breastfed for the first six months of life with continued breastfeeding for two years and beyond.[1] However, there is a colossal difference between saying that you support breastfeeding in that way versus actually doing anything to truly support it. Not only does a policy need a strategy that details how it will be upheld and enabled, but that strategy needs to be implemented rather than simply sitting on the shelf.[2] Areas of need must be identified, resources secured and then targeted towards those areas to make a leap from policy to practice.[3]

Although many in the survey were affected by a lack of funding, the impact on the peer support role was particularly keenly felt. We know how important peer support is in enabling mothers to breastfeed and for longer. It is a core part of grassroots breastfeeding advocacy within communities[4] which is highly valued by women who access it.[5] However, peer support funding had been cut or reduced in many areas meaning that it was a major challenge to keep reliably delivering this much needed service – something that is reflected across the UK and in many countries around the world. This is despite research showing that integration of peer support into health services in a way that allows it to be delivered consistently and equitably is really important.[6]

One of the challenges with breastfeeding funding is that it is often short term, or it is a ring-fenced pot of money to which specific applications need to be made. This is time consuming, can feel inefficient and let's face it, is soul destroying. Wider research shows us that for funding to be truly effective it needs to be sustainable and longer term.[7] Breastfeeding interventions do not work overnight – they take time to embed, complicated by often needing to change broader societal attitudes towards how babies are cared for and fed.[8] Any funding that demands immediate returns rather than focusing on long term societal shifts is going to fall short. Sadly, all too often we see this happen. Short term funding is awarded, key (but impossible) targets are not met, and funding is withdrawn due to a lack of immediate evidence of impact.[9]

Linked to this, when we are measuring breastfeeding 'success' for different interventions we need to consider what that actually looks like. Too frequently it is based only on hard outcome measures e.g. breastfeeding rates, whilst dismissing outcomes that are considered 'softer' such as women's experiences of services and support. However, the issue with relying only on breastfeeding rates is that it takes considerable time for any intervention to make an impact large enough to be considered statistically significant.

We know that breastfeeding is affected by multiple systemic factors. Whilst breastfeeding support from health professionals, lactation specialists and peer supporters works to increase breastfeeding and is valued by mothers,[10] it is only one piece of the jigsaw. Women are still affected by the attitudes and behaviours of family, friends, society, workplaces and industry.[11] Raising breastfeeding rates in any area takes time to create a ripple across that area and 'outcomes' should not be dismissed prematurely without exploring whether any intervention is valued by those it is designed for.

This is a core reason why investment into the wider system is needed and not solely focussed on direct support for mothers. The World Breastfeeding Trends Initiative [WBTI] scores countries on how well they are meeting different aspects that we know support breastfeeding.[12] It measures 10 key indicators including:

1. National policy, programme and coordination. Is there a national infant and young child feeding strategy, a national coordinating committee and a national coordinator, as recommended in the Global Strategy?
2. Baby Friendly Initiative. Do all mothers have access to accredited Baby Friendly maternity care?
3. International Code of Marketing of Breast Milk Substitutes. Are the provisions of the International Code and subsequent World Health Assembly Resolutions (the Code) enacted in national legislation and fully enforced?
4. Maternity protection. Do women have adequate paid maternity leave and breastfeeding breaks?

5. Health professional training. Are all health professionals who work with mothers and babies adequately trained to support breastfeeding?
6. Community-based support. Do all mothers have access to skilled breastfeeding support from health professionals and others in the community?
7. Information support. Is there a comprehensive national information, education and communication strategy, with accurate information on infant and young child feeding at every level?
8. Information support. Is there a comprehensive national information, education and communication strategy, with accurate information on infant and young child feeding at every level?
9. Infant and young child feeding during emergencies. Are guidelines in place to provide protection to infants and young children in case of emergency?
10. Monitoring and evaluation. Are monitoring and evaluation data regularly collected and used to improve infant and young child feeding practices?

Part of this issue is that governments need to refocus resources and energy on tackling the origins of disease. All too often healthcare spending seems to focus on the inevitable health emergencies of systems that do not value health promotion, such as cancer and heart disease, rather than taking a few steps back and investing resources to reduce the levels of non-communicable diseases occurring in the first place.[13] The Heckman curve shows that the strongest return on investments (i.e. the most money saved) comes from investing in the early years of life, infant feeding is a core part of that. However, all too often particularly in high income countries, there is a complete disconnect between understanding the relationship between early feeding experiences and health outcomes.[14]

Within this is a clear need for those working within healthcare and policy organisations to be on board with evidence-based and supportive messaging. It is vitally important that we have strong leadership with everyone 'singing from the same hymn sheet' when it comes to supporting infant feeding. Strong messages 'from above' supports the work of those 'on the ground' working day to day with families.[7] When they can refer to missives and messaging, their work is given further legitimacy.[15]

> *'It would help if our commissioners saw the worth of our work, to have someone in an influential position within the trust who fought for us to provide support.' (IBCLC)*

Feeling supported by those in your field is an integral part of feeling valued in your role. As you have read throughout the book, although many professionals and volunteers gained a lot of strength from supporting families, many felt blocked, criticised and generally undervalued by the broader system. Imagine a world where everyone working in breastfeeding support felt valued by those across the health and social care system? Where their work and expertise was valued and accepted? What a difference that would make to wellbeing, energy and ultimately the families we serve.

Societal change

More broadly than targeting changes to government-led investment is the need to ensure that understanding of the importance of infant feeding is revolutionised across society. If society understood the value of breastfeeding and knew how to support (or simply not block) those who wanted to breastfeed, the job of getting on with the actual support would be much easier. MUCH easier. What did respondents think would help here?

> *'Not being undermined by lack of enforcement of law, the constant level of societal misogyny and lack of honouring of women and feeding at the breast.' (Breastfeeding counsellor)*

As considered in part earlier in this chapter, we know that breastfeeding is part of a complex societal picture. The attitudes of friends, family, employers and even strangers can considerably impact upon the ability of a mother to continue breastfeeding. This is particularly true in areas with very low breastfeeding rates, often considered to be 'formula feeding cultures' where bottle feeding and formula are the norms in terms of behaviour, attitudes and prior experiences. Leading a cultural shift in these areas is extremely challenging, but of course, much needed. Any approach to better supporting breastfeeding that focuses on one aspect alone is unlikely to work well.[7]

Although investing in direct breastfeeding support is important, so too is investment in change across society. Without changes to the culture that surrounds new parents, we will forever be fighting a battle to be that bubble of support. Changes need to focus on the whole system including across perinatal care, a better focus on mental health and normal infant behaviour, upholding maternity and legal rights, preventing predatory breast milk substitute marketing, and educating our broader society about how to protect and support breastfeeding.[11]

Upholding the WHO International Code of Marketing of Breastmilk Substitutes was integral to many responses. Although supporters identified many systemic barriers that stood in the way of accessing good information and support around infant feeding, the underhand and inaccurate messaging and tactics used by the breast milk substitute industry were often central to responses. Frustration at how messages were used to place doubt in mothers and families' minds about the sufficiency and safety of breastfeeding and breast milk was particularly high (and heightened during the pandemic).

'We need adoption and full enforcement of the WHO Code across the land and severe penalties for those who contravene it.' (IBCLC)

'Stopping companies from reaching parents and families would go a long way in making my job easier. I wouldn't have to spend time reassuring, correcting or defending my messaging. It's exhausting.' (Peer supporter)

A central concern related to this was just how much formula had been normalised by advertising and other tactics and was often believed to be the solution to every problem. Formula was often seen as the 'good enough' option and formula companies as supportive and understanding by parents and those who support them.

'Can we have a switch in society from formula being the answer to everything and for women to be more readily able to trust their instincts and bodies.' (Breastfeeding counsellor)

We know that these tactics used by formula companies are deliberate, with carefully constructed messaging to present as a solution to a perceived health or behavioural issue. Relationships with families, especially first-time pregnant women are carefully cultivated with perceptions created that companies are caring and supportive.[16] This leads to parents choosing one brand of formula over another, believing that statements made about health and developmental benefits are 'truthful',[17] when in fact many are inaccurate or lacking in any evidence base.[18]

2.   Changes to breastfeeding support delivery

These recommendations focussed on changes to the way in which breastfeeding support services were delivered. Aside from a simple desire for 'more staff', 'more funding' and 'more peer support groups' to take the strain off a creaking system, or as one breastfeeding counsellor wrote *'More peer supporters to share the load and more health professionals with knowledge of breastfeeding'*, other specific changes were in relation to models of service delivery.

Making changes to the level and quality of support that parents received would directly impact on the day-to-day work and wellbeing across the lactation field as professionals and volunteers would spend less time picking up the pieces of inconsistent, incorrect or absent support and more time focussing on directly supporting families with feeding. With fewer complications to correct, pressure on the broader system would be reduced as many families would not need such intensive support.

As one lactation consultant remarked *'maybe I'm doing myself out of a job here but imagine if no one needed me as a consequence of previously receiving poor professional care??'* So, what would that reimagined system (obviously against a backdrop abundant with funding, supportive senior leadership and societal enthusiasm) look like?

Integrated care with clear referral pathways

One clear area of service development that was identified as needing to receive investment and focus was the importance of having a clear map of what services were in place, and an ability to be able to refer families along them. This had two core elements to it. The first was crucial integration of separate services working in different areas so that they complemented and supported each other. It was clear that there was often a lot of confusion within areas about who was working in different roles and that many different providers were working as separate entities within a system rather than in collaboration with each other. This meant that opportunities for support were missed.

> *'There are lots of different organisations and individuals working in our area which seem a bit piecemeal. I'm not even sure who is who and doing what so how parents are meant to navigate the service I'm not sure. We need to be better organised and work alongside each other rather than presenting in a rather ad hoc and separate way that we do now.' (Health Visitor)*

This lack of integration is likely complex. It might stem from a lack of clear leadership and organisation in an area from the top levels of management. However, it may also be exacerbated by some of the other challenges we have already considered in this book – concerns around securing a share of limited funding, tensions between different professional groups and volunteers and broader struggles with systems and structures that constrain service delivery for some.

This brings us back to the importance of a whole systems approach where every lactation supporter is valued and respected, has access to the training and development they need and most importantly has sufficient funding to deliver the services that they do. At the risk of sounding like a stuck record - without long term investment and engaged leadership, changing any of the other needs can feel like an insurmountable challenge.

The second related issue was for services to be available in the first place. Sometimes practitioners felt that there was simply no option to refer, or a long waiting list or limited service provision.

'It's tough when you know that a mother really needs something such as specialist mental health or tongue tie support or even just a more regular breastfeeding group but a lack of funding means it's not available or she'd have to wait too long.' (GP)

Training across health professional groups

Many respondents in the survey raised the challenge of working within a system where not everyone understood or valued breastfeeding, yet this didn't appear to stop them giving advice to parents. This inability to recognise limitations in knowledge and training, or a belief that breastfeeding didn't matter meant that those working in breastfeeding support often faced an uphill struggle to reverse misinformation before they could get started on solving whatever issue had presented in the first place.

> '*If every single health care professional could do some retraining on breastfeeding and normal infant and child behaviour. Mums don't just come to breastfeeding groups to discuss breastfeeding. Sleep, co-sleeping/bedsharing and slings are also discussed. The amount of GP's and health visitors that offer cry it out or sleep training for infants that just want to be close to their parents is still rife in the area I offer breastfeeding support.' (Peer   supporter)*

This need for joined-up cohesive working has been recognised previously. Interventions only work to their full potential if every professional who encounters a breastfeeding mother knows when to help and when to refer onto another specialist.[19] This of course fits neatly with the previous point around referral pathways. For this to work there obviously needs to be a clear pathway for a professional with less knowledge around supporting breastfeeding to signpost women to.

Unfortunately, this is not a revolutionary finding, many countries find themselves in a position where healthcare staff who have not received training (or sufficient, or updated training) in supporting breastfeeding continue to give misinformation. This can have devastating consequences for a woman's ability to continue breastfeeding and subsequently her mental health. When I wrote 'Why breastfeeding grief and trauma matter' which explores the experiences of those who have been unable to meet their breastfeeding goals, this lack of training, mixed up messaging and misinformation was one of the core issues raised (alongside that lack of referral pathways issue).

At the heart of this is often incorrect information from medical staff, general practitioners and pharmacists who may be looking after other aspects of postnatal health yet have received little training. Many feel uncertain when prescribing medications or procedures[20] and can be overly cautious in a belief that they are protecting infants from potential harmful effects, without taking into consideration the negative implications of breastfeeding cessation. This insecurity is deepened, particularly in the USA, by fears around litigation.[21]

However, for some this is unfortunately driven by a belief that there is little benefit to breastfeeding, particularly after the early weeks.[23] The sad consequence is that breastfeeding often stops prematurely;[24] although in research we led for the Breastfeeding Network, it can also mean that mothers go without necessary medications as they value breastfeeding over their own health issues.[25]

3.   Changes to the breastfeeding supporter role

A core theme that arose throughout the responses was changes that are needed to ensure that more could train, practice and be respected in different breastfeeding supporter roles. The 'workforce' needed greater diversity, flexibility and opportunity across several different aspects of the current set up. These included:

Fair pay and viability of roles

The first suggestion was that investment was needed to ensure that there was less reliance on volunteer roles and that pay reflected the training, skills and investment that went into the role. This did not mean that volunteer posts should disappear as some preferred that option. However, a need for a fairer system of recognition and reward was prominent across global responses:

> *'Fair pay for my work, respect for and understanding of my skills and experience, reliable funding for drop-ins.'* (Breastfeeding counsellor)

> *'If government and [redacted country] doctor association can pay attention to this issue so such as breastfeeding counsellor is not volunteer job anymore.'* (Breastfeeding counsellor)

Changes to training and professional development

Although this idea ties in with the previous discussion around enhanced breastfeeding training across all health care groups, here the focus is placed on opportunities for development for those already within breastfeeding specific roles. Several issues were highlighted here. First, a need for more specialist training for those working within infant feeding specialist roles, particularly for people who had trained before nursing and midwifery courses increased their breastfeeding content.

> 'We need good education programmes for neonatal nurses. I've had two days in ten years but am expected to support mothers with complex feeding issues.' (Neonatal nurse)

Some also felt that those working in management and commissioning didn't understand the value of training and continued professional development for those working in infant feeding roles.

> 'Understanding from the commissioners that breastfeeding training should be a priority for health visitors and support staff and it should be a key performance indicator.' (IBCLC)

Another issue raised was that those who had trained to be an IBCLC but who did not have a healthcare qualification felt that their opportunities were limited. In many hospitals only those with wider nursing skills could apply for infant feeding roles, leaving them only able to set up in private practice.

> 'I only want to give infant feeding support. I don't need wider nursing skills. I can't see me needing to take blood or work a drip so why would I need this training? When I look at job descriptions for infant feeding specialist posts I have all the skills and experience (more if I'm honest than some in these posts) but cannot apply for it because I have not done my general nurse training.' (IBCLC)

This is of course a complex issue. Some posts will require the extensive training that goes alongside a healthcare professional qualification PLUS lactation skills and expertise. However, a more flexible system that took into account expertise and role requirements would help to integrate roles. Potentially, additional training for those wishing to work within hospital systems may be another solution, akin to UK midwifery 18-month (compared with 3 year) training courses for those with existing healthcare qualifications. Could a training course be developed to enhance the clinical skills of those in IBCLC roles who have not yet undertaken healthcare professional training?

Surely working more closely together would also help each professional recognise their strengths and knowledge gaps (i.e. in lactation or clinical skills) and learn from each other, taking the lead on areas of expertise, but also fostering greater collaboration and interprofessional working. At the least this conversation needs taking further forward.

Enhanced collaborative working

Recognition of the strength and contribution across all roles and enhanced ways to work collaboratively together was another core recommendation. Although each qualification / role has supporting breastfeeding and families at its heart, there are distinct differences that work well in combination. Although different qualifications may represent different training and skills this shouldn't be viewed as a hierarchy but rather complementary skills and focus. Yes of course complex cases require a practitioner with advanced training but that doesn't mean that peer support doesn't play its role. Finding that balance is the challenge.

'Recognition from healthcare professionals (ie GPs and health visitors) that breastfeeding counsellors actually provide a hugely valuable service, and in fact are knowledgeable!' (Breastfeeding counsellor)

More accessible mentoring and wellbeing support

It's hopefully a no-brainer after reading this book that there needs to be better support pathways in place for those working in the field of lactation. Participants identified that this needed to include a whole spectrum of support from productive mentoring sessions that really drove development and reflection, to support structures around those who were struggling with their mental health. In terms of mentoring and supervision, there are clear gaps and a need for more of this support, particularly for those newly qualified as lactation consultants. Many desired and would value being able to turn to someone more experienced in the field for advice and mentorship.

'I would very much value having someone to debrief with more regularly. At the moment I rely on trusted peers, often daily if you consider offloading all my frustrations to be a debrief. My peers are wonderful but have their own struggles. I would jump at the opportunity to have more structured debrief opportunities from someone trained to do this.' (IBCLC)

For those in employed or peer support positions, while many noted that they could always turn to a supervisor for support, they felt that they needed more input and time than was available. Most recognised that this was due to time pressures and part of the larger picture of services being underfunded and resourced, yet again highlighting the bottom line need for sustained investment in services.

'My line manager is amazing and always has time for me if I need her but sometimes I worry that I'm putting too much on her. She is so busy and trying to keep the service running. I know it's important that I seek supervision but sometimes I hold back as I think that when she's spending time with me, she's not spending time with a complex case or something that would benefit more families.' (Midwife).

171

Investment in diversity and the future

Last but very much not least, a core issue raised was the vital need to think about the future of the lactation workforce, both in terms of succession planning and diversity. Several respondents with many decades of experience were very aware that they would be retiring or unable to support families in the future and were concerned about the loss of that knowledge and skill alongside no clear definitive plans to replace it.

> 'A big part of the midwifery crisis is to do with the age of the workforce. Many of my colleagues and I will be retiring in 10 years. If they don't start to contingency plan there will be no one to take our places.' (Infant feeding lead)

A second issue was the lack of diversity in the professional and volunteer space. As explored in earlier chapters some supporters, especially those who felt unable to train as IBCLCs, did not feel accepted or represented in the profession. This included aspects such as age, ethnicity, education, neurodiversity and LGBTQ identity. In all cases participants felt excluded because of difference. For some this intersected with financial, cultural or experiential difficulties making training much more difficult.

> 'Breastfeeding is universal but the supporters that I are not. Where is the visibility and diversity? Are we giving the impression that only a certain type of woman breastfeeds because we know that's not what we're about but might inadvertently be saying. Who aren't we reaching because we didn't bring more women on board?' (Peer supporter)

> 'There are still major barriers to who becomes an IBCLC, who sets up in professional practice and who makes money. The people doing this successfully do not fully reflect the communities that they serve and this needs to change. They are great colleagues but we need to bring more people on board, we need to grow and expand.' (IBCLC)

The issue of barriers to training is important on multiple levels. It goes without saying that it is critical from a diversity and inclusion perspective, but also matters in terms of representing the families that we serve. If individuals are facing barriers to even accessing training and development in the first place, it is no wonder that we see a lack of diversity in leadership positions in organisations, in well-paid roles and representing the profession. We hear about the 'leaky pipeline' when it comes to women in the workplace i.e. women dropping out of work or leadership tracks due to structural issues and attitudes. The same is true across all intersections and aspects of the lactation field.

Greater investment is needed in supporting initiatives that specifically open up training opportunities for those from under-represented and historically excluded groups. There are growing organisations now offering bespoke training to tackle inequalities in training from a racial and ethnicity perspective. To illustrate this, two I will draw attention to are the Indigenous Lactation Counselor training course that is Native owned, designed and taught, and is specifically for those that identify as Indigenous. Find them @IndigenousLactationCounselor on Facebook. Likewise, the Blacktavist peer counselor training programme is aimed at aspiring Black lactation professionals and Non-Black Allies supporting Black Communities. Find them at https://theblackcourse.com.

For more initiatives, context and reflection, La Leche League GB has collated a brilliant list of resources led by Black and Brown expert voices entitled 'In pursuit of equitable breastfeeding support' with articles and recordings by experts in racial disparities and exclusion around birth and infant feeding, including Kimberly Seals Allers, Nekisha Killings, and Ruth Dennison. You can find it at https://www.laleche.org.uk/in-pursuit-of-equitable-breastfeeding-support/.

Similar investment is needed in expanding training opportunities to reduce other disparities, such as those from a LGBTQ, neurodiversity and disability perspective. Although initiatives to reduce socioeconomic inequalities are more common to allow those in less affluent neighbourhoods to train as peer supporters, or discounts are available for some courses or training based on income, this solves only part of the issue.

From survey responses it is clear that it is not just support for more to access training opportunities in the first place that is required. Clearly investment is needed to remove the structural and systemic barriers that prevent people from being able to make a living from lactation support and to continue with training and development once qualified. Likewise, who gets to progress in management or research positions? Funding to enable peer supporter training or an IBCLC application for example is so important but what then?

We need an overhaul of the whole systems and structure around lactation support. More bursaries and subsidies, yes. But also more opportunity for defined career paths, banishing shame around charging our worth, mentoring and career coaching opportunities, and bigger societal changes such as business start-up funding, more affordable childcare and flexible working. Basically, every barrier that has been discussed in this book needs viewing through an intersectional lens, particularly as those barriers hit ten times harder when you're starting from a place of inequity.

Coming back full circle, of course this lack of opportunity and support is part of the bigger issue of a government and society that doesn't value or support infant feeding in the first place. We will never see central funding and investment in moving things forward until we see lactation support and breastfeeding valued as the critical early influence that it is. Until then, keep fighting. Remember your worth and the value of what we are striving for. And just as importantly, never forget to treat yourself with the same kindness, respect and compassion as the families that you support and care for.

Chapter 10

Further resources

Finally, here are some further resources that can support you with exploring your mental health and learning more about burnout, stress and the broader context of working within lactation support. First, there are some excellent recordings available from IBCLC specialising in supporting the wellbeing of their colleagues. I have included links to available recordings (many available from Gold Leaning). These include:

- **Nekisha Killings**: Approaching Care When You're Barely There: Reimagining Empathy When You've Got Nothing Left to Give
  https://www.goldlearning.com/lecture/1527

- **Dr Kathy Kendall Tackett**: Burnout, Compassion Fatigue and Self-Care for Members of the Perinatal Team https://www.goldlearning.com/lecture/158

- **Annie Frisbie and Leah Jolly:** Compassion Fatigue and the Lactation Consultant
  https://paperlesslactation.com/blog/compassion-fatigue-and-the-ibclc-podcast/

Further reading

Here are some further books (in alphabetical order) that you may like around the concepts of burnout, supporting wellbeing and broader influences on infant feeding:

- Breastfeeding Uncovered: Who really decides how we feed our babies - Amy Brown
- Covid Babies: How pandemic health measures undermined pregnancy, birth and early parenting – Amy Brown

- Daring Greatly: How the courage to be vulnerable transforms the way we live, love, parent and lead – Brené Brown
- Keep The Fires Burning: Conquering stress and burnout as a Mother-Baby Professional - Micky Jones
- Nurturing Maternity Staff: How to tackle trauma, stress and burnout to create a positive working culture in the NHS - Jan Smith
- The Big Letdown: How Medicine, Big Business, and Feminism Undermine Breastfeeding - Kimberly Seals Allers
- The gifts of imperfection: Let go of who you think you're supposed to be and embrace who you are - Brené Brown
- The Joy of Burnout: How the end of the world can be a new beginning - Dina Glouberman
- The politics of breastfeeding - Gabrielle Palmer
- Unlatched: The Evolution of Breastfeeding and the Making of a Controversy - Jennifer Grayson
- Why Breastfeeding Grief and Trauma matter - Amy Brown

Mental health resources

If you are struggling with your mental health please do speak to your GP or doctor. However, there are some good places that you can also go for support. I apologise that these are UK centric and I cannot list resources for every country - although many of these websites have articles and resources that are relevant from a global perspective.

- NHS Every Mind Matters https://www.nhs.uk/every-mind-matters
- Mind https://www.mind.org.uk
- The Samaritans https://www.samaritans.org
- Welldoing https://welldoing.org

References

Introduction
1. How did US baby formula get contaminated with dangerous bacteria? New Scientist 17.05.22
2. Hall LH et al. Healthcare staff wellbeing, burnout, and patient safety: a systematic review. PloS one. 2016 Jul 8;11(7):e0159015.
3. Suleiman-Martos N et al. Prevalence and predictors of burnout in midwives: a systematic review and meta-analysis. International journal of environmental research and public health. 2020;17(2):641.
4. Khamisa N et al. Work related stress, burnout, job satisfaction and general health of nurses. International journal of environmental research and public health. 2015 Jan;12(1):652-66.
5. Brown A. What do women lose if they are prevented from meeting their breastfeeding goals?. Clinical Lactation. 2018 Nov 1;9(4):200-7.

Chapter 1: Joy & burnout in the lactation field
1. McFadden A et al. Support for healthy breastfeeding mothers with healthy term babies. Cochrane Database of Systematic Reviews. 2017(2).
2. Hunter, B., 2010. Mapping the emotional terrain of midwifery: what can we see and what lies ahead?. *International Journal of Work Organisation and Emotion*, 3(3), pp.253-269.
3. Shakespeare J et al. How do women with postnatal depression experience listening visits in primary care? A qualitative interview study. JRIP. 2006; 24:149-62.
4. Taylor J et al. A hermeneutic phenomenological study exploring the experience health practitioners have when working with families to safeguard children and the invisibility of the emotions work involved. Journal of Clinical Nursing. 2017 Feb;26(3-4):557-67.
5. Bria M et al. Systematic review of burnout risk factors among European healthcare professionals. Cognition, Brain, Behavior: An Interdisciplinary Journal. 2012 1;16(3):423-52.
6. Reed A. Overdue: Birth, burnout and a blueprint for a better NHS. 2020. Pinter & Martin Ltd.
7. Graham C. 'Why are burnout and poor working experiences so common among midwives?' Nursing Times 23.05.22
8. Mollart L et al. Midwives' emotional wellbeing: impact of conducting a structured antenatal psychosocial assessment. Women and Birth. 2009 Sep 1;22(3):82-8.
9. Knight M, Stanford S. Ockenden: another shocking review of maternity services. bmj. 2022 Apr 6;377.
10. RCM (2021) RCM warns of midwife exodus as maternity staffing crisis grows. Accessed via: https://www.rcm.org.uk/media-releases/2021/september/rcm-warns-of-midwife-exodus-as-maternity-staffing-crisis-grows/

11. IHV 2020 https://ihv.org.uk/news-and-views/news/health-visitors-fear-for-childrens-wellbeing-due-to-relentless-service-cuts/

12. IHV 2021 State of Health Visiting in England https://ihv.org.uk/wp-content/uploads/2021/11/State-of-Health-Visiting-Survey-2021-FINAL-VERSION-25.11.21.pdf

13. GMC (2021) Doctors' burnout worsens as GMC report reveals pandemic impact. https://www.gmc-uk.org/news/news-archive/doctors-burnout-worsens-as-gmc-report-reveals-pandemic-impact

14. https://www.theguardian.com/society/2020/jan/27/third-of-uk-doctors-report-burnout-and-compassion-fatigue

15. McKinley N et al. Resilience, burnout and coping mechanisms in UK doctors: a cross-sectional study. BMJ open. 2020; 1;10(1):031765.

16. Britten, J., Hoddinott, P., & McInnes, R. (2006). Breastfeeding peer support: health service programmes in Scotland. *BJM*, *14*(1), 12-19.

17. Hopper, H. and Skirton, H., 2016. Factors influencing the sustainability of volunteer peer support for breast-feeding mothers within a hospital environment: An exploratory qualitative study. *Midwifery*, *32*, pp.58-65.

18. Curtis P et al. The peer-professional interface in a community-based, breastfeeding peer-support project. 2007. *Midwifery*, *23*(2), pp.146-156.

19. Ward, L.P., Williamson, S., Burke, S., Crawford-Hemphill, R. and Thompson, A.M., 2017. Improving exclusive breastfeeding in an urban academic hospital. *Pediatrics*, *139*(2).

20. Hunter B et al. Midwives in the United Kingdom: Levels of burnout, depression, anxiety and stress and associated predictors. 2019l; *Midwifery*, *79*, p.102526.

21. Creedy DK, Sidebotham M, Gamble J, Pallant J, Fenwick J. Prevalence of burnout, depression, anxiety and stress in Australian midwives: a cross-sectional survey. BMC pregnancy and childbirth. 2017 Dec;17(1):1-8.

22. Maharaj S et al. Prevalence and risk factors of depression, anxiety, and stress in a cohort of Australian nurses. International journal of environmental research and public health. 2019 Jan;16(1):61.

23. Cheung T, Yip PS. Depression, anxiety and symptoms of stress among Hong Kong nurses: a cross-sectional study. IJERPH. 2015 Sep;12(9):11072-100.

24. Prasad K et al. Prevalence and correlates of stress and burnout among US healthcare workers during the COVID-19 pandemic: A national cross-sectional survey study. EClinicalMedicine. 2021; 1;35:100879.

25. Hope V, Henderson M. Medical student depression, anxiety and distress outside N orth A merica: a systematic review. Medical education. 2014 Oct;48(10):963-79.

26. Marvaldi M et al. Anxiety, depression, trauma-related, and sleep disorders among healthcare workers during the COVID-19

pandemic: A systematic review and meta-analysis. Neuroscience & Biobehavioral Reviews. 2021 Jul 1;126:252-64.

27. Maslach C, Jackson SE. The measurement of experienced burnout. Journal of organizational behavior. 1981 Apr;2(2):99-113.

28. ICD11 https://www.who.int/news/item/28-05-2019-burn-out-an-occupational-phenomenon-international-classification-of-diseases

29. Tucker SJ, Weymiller AJ, Cutshall SM, Rhudy LM, Lohse CM. Stress ratings and health promotion practices among RNs: a case for action. J Nurs Adm 2012; 42: 282-92.

30. Maslach, C. (1982). Burnout: The cost of caring. Englewood Cliffs, New Jersey: Prentice Hall.

31. Koutsimani P, Montgomery A, Georganta K. The relationship between burnout, depression, and anxiety: A systematic review and meta-analysis. Frontiers in psychology. 2019 Mar 13;10:284.

32. Laschinger HK, Grau AL. The influence of personal dispositional factors and organizational resources on workplace violence, burnout, and health outcomes in new graduate nurses: A cross-sectional study. IJNS. 2012; 1;49(3):282-91.

33. Da Silva RM et al. Hardy personality and burnout syndrome among nursing students in three Brazilian universities -an analytic study. BMC Nurs 2014; 13: 9.

34. Young CM, Smythe L, Couper JM. Burnout: Lessons from the lived experience of case loading midwives. International Journal of Childbirth. 2015 Jan 1;5(3):154-65.

35. Brown A. Why breastfeeding grief and trauma matter. 2019. Pinter and Martin Ltd.

36. Joinson C. Coping with compassion fatigue. Nursing. 1992 Apr 1;22(4):116-8.

37. Cohen S, Janicki-Deverts D, Miller GE. Psychological stress and disease. Jama. 2007 Oct 10;298(14):1685-7.

38. Figley CR. Compassion fatigue: Psychotherapists' chronic lack of self care. Journal of clinical psychology. 2002 Nov;58(11):1433-41.

39. Coetzee S, Klopper H. Compassion fatigue within nursing practice: A concept analysis. Nursing & health sciences. 2010;12(2):235-43.

40. Fernando III AT, Consedine NS. Beyond compassion fatigue: the transactional model of physician compassion. Journal of pain and symptom management. 2014 Aug 1;48(2):289-98.

41. Huggard P. Caring for the carers: compassion fatigue and disenfranchised grief. In Science with feeling: animals and people. Australia and Royal Society of New Zealand Anzccart Conference Proceedings 2016 (Vol. 28).

42. Baranowsky AB. The silencing response in clinical practice: On the road to dialogue. Treating compassion fatigue. 2002 Jun 28:155-70.

43. Kumar S. Burnout and doctors: prevalence, prevention and intervention. InHealthcare 2016 Sep (Vol. 4, No. 3, p. 37). Multidisciplinary Digital Publishing Institute.

44. Khamisa N, Peltzer K, Oldenburg B. Burnout in relation to specific contributing factors and health outcomes among nurses: a systematic review. IJERPH. 2013 Jun;10(6):2214-40.
45. Naiman-Sessions M, Henley MM, Roth LM. Bearing the burden of care: emotional burnout among maternity support workers. In Health and health care concerns among women and racial and ethnic minorities 2017 Aug 10. Emerald Publishing Limited.
46. https://gdc.unicef.org/resource/why-women-are-more-burned-out-men
47. Beauregard N et al. Gendered pathways to burnout: results from the SALVEO study. AWEH. 2018 18;62(4):426-37.
48. Villwock J et al. Harris. Imposter syndrome and burnout among American medical students: A pilot study. 2016 *IJME*. 7:364-369.
49. Guille C et al. Work-family conflict and the sex difference in depression among training physicians. 2017. *JAMA Internal Medicine* 177(12):1766-1772.
50. Sinclair S et al. Compassion fatigue: A meta-narrative review of the healthcare literature. IJNS. 2017 1;69:9-24.
51. Cho HJ, Jung MS. Effect of empathy, resilience, self-care on compassion fatigue in oncology nurses. Journal of Korean Academy of Nursing Administration. 2014 1;20(4):373-82.
52. Kendall-Tackett K. Caring for Ourselves When Caring for Others: What Lactation Consultants Need to Know About Compassion Fatigue. Clinical Lactation. 2013 1;4(4):137-8.
53. Dodgson JE. The Pandemic Has Brought Too Much Change: Too Many Preprints; Too Many Retractions. JHL. 2022 May;38(2):207-8.
54. Altman D. Lactation Care of Families in the Community Health Setting During the COVID Pandemic. Clinical Lactation. 2020 25;11(4):185-8.
55. Kristensen T et al. The Copenhagen Burnout Inventory: A new tool for the assessment of burnout. Work & stress. 2005, 1;19(3):192-207.
56. Jordan K et al. Level of burnout in a small population of Australian midwives. Women and Birth. 2013 Jun 1;26(2):125-32.
57. Hildingsson, I., Westlund, K., & Wiklund, I. (2013). Burnout in Swedish midwives. Sexual & Reproductive Healthcare, 4(3), 87-91.

Chapter 2 The impact of working in a system that doesn't value or support breastfeeding

1. Brown A. Breastfeeding Uncovered: Who really decides how we feed our babies? 2021. Second edition. Pinter & Martin Ltd.
2. Regan, S., & Brown, A. (2019). Experiences of online breastfeeding support: Support and reassurance versus judgement and misinformation. *Maternal & Child Nutrition*, 15(4), e12874.
3. Lefebvre C et al. Social media usage among nurses: perceptions and practices. JONA.2020, 1; 50:135-41.
4. Islam A et al. Does multitasking computer self-efficacy mitigate the impact of social media affordances on overload & fatigue among professionals? Information Technology & People. 2020; 34:1439–61.

5.   Morse H, Brown A. Using Facebook groups to support families: midwives' perceptions and experiences of professional social media use. medRxiv. 2022 Jan 1.

6.   Cooper, C.R., 2021. *Super-Natural Breastfeeding: How Lactation Consultants in Hawai 'i Demedicalize and Reshape Women's Embodied Experiences* (Doctoral dissertation, University of Hawai'i at Manoa).

7.   Scarpello, T et al. A qualitative assessment of using lay trainers with type 2 diabetes in an intervention programme for people at risk of type 2 diabetes. 2013, *Health Education Journal*, 72(1), pp.86-94.

8.   Brown A. What do women really want? Lessons for breastfeeding promotion and education. Breastfeeding medicine. 2016, 1;11:102-10.

9.   Hocking J. Managing Connection and Disconnection: relationships as the centre of Lactation Consultant care for breastfeeding women and their babies. A thesis submitted to Western Sydney University.

10. https://www.laleche.hokorg.uk/the-history-of-la-leche-league-celebrating-two-milestone-anniversaries-in-2021/

11. https://www.independent.co.uk/news/science/pms-erectile-dysfunction-studies-penis-problems-period-pre-menstrual-pains-science-disparity-a7198681.html

12. NHS England (2016) National maternity review. better births; improving outcomes of maternity services in England.

13. https://www.irishtimes.com/business/health-pharma/dublin-based-coroflo-gets-richard-branson-s-approval-raises-650-000-1.3260509

14. https://edition.cnn.com/2022/05/03/business/lab-grown-human-milk-biomilq-health-climate-hnk-spc-intl/index.html

15. World Health Organization. (2022) How the marketing of formula milk   influences   our   decisions   on   infant   feeding. https://apps.who.int/iris/bitstream/handle/10665/352098/9789240044609-eng.pdf?sequence=1

16. https://www.nekishakillings.com/speaking-coaching

17. Brown A. Informed is best. How to spot fake news about your pregnancy, birth and baby. 2019. Pinter & Martin.

18. Hakim C. Women, careers, and work-life preferences. British Journal of Guidance & Counselling. 2006, 1;34(3):279-94.

19. Seedat S, Rondon M. Women's wellbeing and the burden of unpaid work. bmj. 2021 Aug 31;374.

20. Hochschild, A. (1989) The Second Shift: Working Parents and the Revolution at Home. New York: Penguin.

21. Mayrhofer W et al. The influence of family responsibilities, career fields and gender on career success. 2008. JMP, 23,3, 292–323.

22. Maher J. Women's care/career changes as connection and resilience: Challenging discourses of breakdown and conflict. Gender, Work & Organization. 2013 Mar;20(2):172-83.

Chapter 3. Passion, empathy & our challenging feeding experiences

1.   Petrucci C et al. Empathy in health professional students: A comparative cross-sectional study. Nurse education. 2016, 1;41:1-5.

2. Moloney S, Gair S. Empathy and spiritual care in midwifery practice: Contributing to women's enhanced birth experiences. Women and Birth. 2015 Dec 1;28(4):323-8.

3. Caelli K et al. Parents' experiences of midwife-managed care following the loss of a baby in a previous pregnancy. JAN. 2002 ;39(2):127-36.

4. Turner KM, Chew-Graham C, Folkes L, Sharp D. Women's experiences of health visitor delivered listening visits as a treatment for postnatal depression: a qualitative study. Patient education and counseling. 2010 Feb 1;78(2):234-9.

5. Emmott EH, Page AE, Myers S. Typologies of postnatal support and breastfeeding at two months in the UK. SSM. 2020 Feb 1;246:112791.

6. Blixt I et al. Women's advice to healthcare professionals regarding breastfeeding:"offer sensitive individualized breastfeeding support"-an interview study. IBJ. 2019 Dec;14(1):1-2.

7. Copeland L et al. Feasibility and acceptability of a motivational interviewing breastfeeding peer support intervention. Maternal & Child Nutrition. 2019 Apr;15(2):e12703.

8. Chang Y et al. Views and experiences of women, peer supporters and healthcare professionals on breastfeeding peer support: A systematic review of qualitative studies. Midwifery. 2022, 1:103299.

9. Rothschild, B., 2006. *Help for the helper: The psychophysiology of compassion fatigue and vicarious trauma.* WW Norton & Company.

10. Sheen, K., Slade, P., & Spiby, H. (2014). An integrative review of the impact of indirect trauma exposure in health professionals and potential issues of salience for midwives. JAN, 70(4), 729–743.

11. Ferri, P., Guerra, E., Marcheselli, L., Cunico, L. and Di Lorenzo, R., 2015. Empathy and burnout: an analytic cross-sectional study among nurses and nursing students.

12. Gleichgerrcht E, Decety J. The costs of empathy among health professionals. In: Decety J, editor. Empathy: from Bench to Bedside. Cambridge: MIT Press; 2012.

13. Stebnicki, M. (2008). Empathy fatigue: Healing the mind, body, and spirit of professional counselors. New York, NY: Springer.

14. Moudatsou M et al. The role of empathy in health and social care professionals. In Healthcare 2020 Mar (Vol. 8, No. 1, p. 26). Multidisciplinary Digital Publishing Institute.

15. Hocking J. Managing Connection and Disconnection: relationships as the centre of Lactation Consultant care for breastfeeding women and their babies. A thesis submitted to Western Sydney University.

16. Jolliffe, D., & Farrington, D. P. (2006). Development and validation of the Basic Empathy Scale. *Journal of adolescence, 29*(4), 589-611.

17. Carré, A et al. The Basic Empathy Scale in adults: factor structure of a revised form. 2013. *Psychological assessment, 25*(3), p.679.

18. Hopper H, Skirton, H. Factors influencing the sustainability of peer support for breast-feeding mothers within a hospital environment: An exploratory qualitative study. 2016. *Midwifery, 32*, pp.58-65.

19. Brown A. Why breastfeeding grief and trauma matter. 2019. Pinter & Martin Ltd.

20. Brown A, Rance J, Bennett P. Understanding the relationship between breastfeeding and postnatal depression: the role of pain and physical difficulties. JAN. 2016 Feb;72(2):273-82.

21. Taylor EN, Wallace LE. For shame: Feminism, breastfeeding advocacy, and maternal guilt. Hypatia. 2012;27(1):76-98.

22. Brown A. What do women lose if they are prevented from meeting their breastfeeding goals?. Clinical Lactation. 2018 Nov 1;9(4):200-7.

23. Burns, E. and Schmied, V., 2017. "The right help at the right time": Positive constructions of peer and professional support for breastfeeding. *Women and Birth, 30*(5), pp.389-397.

24. Thelwell, E., Rheeston, M. and Douglas, H., 2017. Exploring breastfeeding peer supporters' experiences of using the Solihull Approach model. *British Journal of Midwifery, 25*(10), pp.639-646.

25. Britten, J., Hoddinott, P., & McInnes, R. (2006). Breastfeeding peer support: health service programmes in Scotland. *British Journal of Midwifery, 14*(1), 12-19.

26. Chang YS, Beake MS, Kam MJ, Lok KY, Bick D. Views and experiences of women, peer supporters and healthcare professionals on breastfeeding peer support: A systematic review of qualitative studies. Midwifery. 2022 Mar 1:103299.

27. Waggoner, M. Monitoring milk and motherhood: Lactation Consultants and the Dilemmas of Breastfeeding Advocacy. 2011. *International Journal of Sociology of the Family, 37*(1), 153-171.

28. Pearlman, L. A., & Saakvitne, K. W. (1995). Trauma and the therapist: Countertransference and vicarious traumatization in psychotherapy with incest survivors. Norton

29. Newell JM, MacNeil GA. Professional burnout, vicarious trauma, secondary traumatic stress, and compassion fatigue. Best practices in mental health. 2010 Jul 1;6(2):57-68.

30. Kendall-Tackett K, Beck CT. Secondary Traumatic Stress and Moral Injury in Maternity Care Providers: A Narrative and Exploratory Review. Frontiers in Global Women's Health. 2022;3.

31. Elmir, R., Schmied, V., Wilkes, L., & Jackson, D. (2010). Women's perceptions and experiences of a traumatic birth: A meta-ethnography. Journal of Advanced Nursing, 66(10), 2142–2153.

32. Schrøder K et al. Guilt without fault: A qualitative study into the ethics of forgiveness after traumatic childbirth. 2017. Social Science & Medicine, 176, 14–20.

33. Shorey, S. and Wong, P.Z.E., 2021. Vicarious Trauma Experienced by Health Care Providers Involved in Traumatic Childbirths: A Meta-Synthesis. *Trauma, Violence, & Abuse,* p.15248380211013135.

34. Rice, H., & Warland, J. (2013). Bearing witness: Midwives experiences of witnessing traumatic birth. Midwifery, 29, 1056–1063.

35. Lawton K. Midwives' experiences of helping women struggling to breastfeed. 2016. *British Journal of Healthcare Assistants, 10*(6),270-275.

36. Toohill, J., Fenwick, J., Sidebotham, M., Gamble, J., & Creedy, D. K. (2019). Trauma and fear in Australian midwives. Women and Birth, 32(1), 64–71. https://doi.org/10.1016/j.wombi.2018.04.003

37. Coldridge, L., & Davies, S. (2017). "Am I too emotional for this job?" an exploration of student midwives' experiences of coping with traumatic events in the labour ward. Midwifery, 45, 1–6.

38. Mezey G et al. Midwives' perceptions and experiences of routine enquiry for domestic violence. BJOG: an international journal of obstetrics and gynaecology. 2003 Aug 1;110(8):744-52.

Chapter 4: The stress of disconnection and conflict

1. Rossman B et al. Healthcare providers' perceptions of breastfeeding peer counselors in the neonatal intensive care unit. *Research in nursing & health*, 2012, 35, pp.460-474.

2. Thomson G et al. Building social capital through breastfeeding peer support: insights from an evaluation of a voluntary breastfeeding peer support service in North-West England. *IBJ*, 2015, 10(1).1-14.

3. Ingram J. A mixed methods evaluation of peer support in Bristol, UK: mothers', midwives' and peer supporters' views and the effects on breastfeeding. BMC pregnancy and childbirth. 2013;13(1):1-0.

4. Aiken, A. and Thomson, G., 2013. Professionalisation of a breast-feeding peer support service: issues and experiences of peer supporters. *Midwifery*, 29(12), pp.e145-e151.

5. Oriel K, Plane MB, Mundt M. Family medicine residents and the impostor phenomenon. Fam Med. 2004;36:248–252.

6. Legassie J, Zibrowski EM, Goldszmidt MA. Measuring resident well-being: impostorism and burnout syndrome in residency. J Gen Intern Med. 2008;23:1090–1094

7. LaDonna KA, Ginsburg S, Watling C. "Rising to the level of your incompetence": what physicians' self-assessment of their performance reveals about the imposter syndrome in medicine. Acad Med. 2018;93(5):763–768.

8. Villwock JA, Sobin LB, Koester LA, Harris TM. Impostor syndrome and burnout among American medical students: a pilot study. Int J Med Educ. 2016;7:364–369.

9. Crawford WS, Shanine KK, Whitman MV, et al. Examining the impostor phenomenon and work-family conflict. Journal of Managerial Psychology. 2016; 31(2): 375-390.

10. Wilson JL. An exploration of bullying behaviours in nursing: a review of the literature. BJN. 2016 Mar 24;25(6):303-6.

11. Meissner J (1986) Nurses Are we eating out young? Nursing 16, 51-3

12. Becher J., Visovsky C. (2012) Horizontal Violence in Nursing Medsurg Nursing 21(4) 210-232

13. Rodwell J, Demir D. Psychological Consequences of Bullying for Hospital and Aged Care Homes. INR, 2012, 59 539-546

14. Murray J. (2009) Workplace Bullying in Nursing: A problem that can't be Ignored. Medsurg Nursing 18(5) 273-276

15. Sauer P. (2012) Do Nurses Eat Their Young? Truth and Consequences. Journal of Emergency Nursing 38(1) 43-46

16. Sousa M. (2012) Management and Leadership: The Elephant in the Room; The Truth about Bullying in Nursing Journal of Radiology Nursing 31(1) 29-31

17. Young CM, Smythe L, Couper JM. Burnout: Lessons from the lived experience of case loading midwives. International Journal of Childbirth. 2015 Jan 1;5(3):154-65.

18. Glasper A. Protecting healthcare staff from abuse: tackling workplace incivility in nursing. British journal of nursing. 2018 Dec 13;27(22):1336-7.

19. Wilkins J. The use of cognitive reappraisal and humour as coping strategies for bullied nurses. International journal of nursing practice. 2014 Jun;20(3):283-92.

20. Brown A, Shenker N. Experiences of breastfeeding during COVID-19: Lessons for future practical and emotional support. Maternal & child nutrition. 2021 Jan;17(1):e13088.

21. Hull N, Kam RL, Gribble KD. Providing breastfeeding support during the COVID-19 pandemic: Concerns of mothers who contacted the Australian Breastfeeding Association. Breastfeeding Review. 2020 Nov;28(3):25-35.

22. Robinson A et al. It takes an e-village: Supporting African American mothers in sustaining breastfeeding through Facebook communities. JHL 2019, 35(3), 569–582.

23. Skelton K et al. Exploring social media group use among breastfeeding mothers: Qualitative analysis. JMIR Pediatrics and Parenting. 2018, 1(2), e11344.

24. Black, R et al (2020). Women's experience of social media breastfeeding support and its impact on extended breastfeeding success: A social cognitive perspective. BJHP, 25(3), 754–771.

25. Regan S, Brown A. Experiences of online breastfeeding support: Support and reassurance versus judgement and misinformation. Maternal & Child Nutrition. 2019 Oct;15(4):e12874.

26. Bridges N et al. Exploring breastfeeding support on social media. International Breastfeeding Journal, 2018, 13(1), 22

27. Horan G. Feminazi, breastfeeding nazi, grammar nazi. A critical analysis of nazi insults in contemporary media discourses. Mediazioni. 2019;24.

28. Staricka C. Lactivism: How Feminists and Fundamentalists, Hippies and Yuppies, and Physicians and Politicians Made Breastfeeding Big Business and Bad Policy. Clinical Lactation. 2016;7(2):79.

Chapter 5: Financial pressures and privilege

1. Thompson R et al. An account of significant events influencing Australian breastfeeding practice over the last 40 years. Women and Birth. 2011 Sep 1;24(3):97-104.

2. Aiken, A. and Thomson, G., 2013. Professionalisation of a breast-feeding peer support service: issues and experiences of peer supporters. *Midwifery, 29*(12), pp.e145-e151.
3. Britten J et al. Breastfeeding peer support: health service programmes in Scotland. *BJM*, 2006, *14*(1), 12-19.
4. Grant A et al. Autistic women's views & experiences of infant feeding: A systematic review of qualitative evidence. Autism. 2022 12:13623613221089374.

Chapter 6: The impact of the Covid-19 pandemic

1. Renfrew, M et al.. Sustaining quality midwifery care in a pandemic and beyond. Midwifery. 2020 Sep;88:102759.
2. Brown A, Shenker N. Breastfeeding support during COVID-19. 2020. Accessed via https://www.breastfeedingnetwork.org.uk/wp-content/uploads/2020/08/BFN-Summary-COVID.pdf
3. Hull N, Kam RL, Gribble KD. Providing breastfeeding support during the COVID-19 pandemic: Concerns of mothers who contacted the ABA. Breastfeeding Review. 2020 Nov;28(3):25-35.
4. Brown A, Shenker N. Experiences of breastfeeding during COVID-19: Lessons for future practical and emotional support. Maternal & child nutrition. 2021 Jan;17(1):e13088.
5. Best Beginnings et al. Babies in Lockdown report. 2020. Access via www.babiesinlockdown.info
6. Snyder K, Worlton G. Social support during COVID-19: perspectives of breastfeeding mothers. Breastfeeding Medicine. 2021 Jan 1;16(1):39-45.
7. Turner S et al. A review of the disruption of breastfeeding supports in response to the COVID-19 pandemic in five Western countries and applications for clinical practice. IBJ. 2022;17(1):1-3.
8. Vassilopoulou E et al. Breastfeeding and COVID-19: from nutrition to immunity. Frontiers in immunology. 2021 Apr 7;12:946.
9. https://www.who.int/news-room/commentaries/detail/breastfeeding-and-covid-19
10. IHV 2021 State of Health Visiting in England https://ihv.org.uk/wp-content/uploads/2021/11/State-of-Health-Visiting-Survey-2021-FINAL-VERSION-25.11.21.pdf
11. Aksoy YE, Koçak V. Psychological effects of nurses and midwives due to COVID-19 outbreak: The case of Turkey. Archives of psychiatric nursing. 2020 Oct 1;34(5):427-33.
12. Conti G, Dow A. The impacts of COVID-19 on Health Visiting Services in England: FOI Evidence for the First Wave. Accessed via https://discovery.ucl.ac.uk/id/eprint/10122752/
13. Panda PK et al. Psychological and behavioral impact of lockdown and quarantine measures for COVID-19 pandemic on children, adolescents and caregivers: a systematic review and meta-analysis. Journal of tropical pediatrics. 2021 Feb;67(1):fmaa122.

14. Sanders J, Blaylock R. "Anxious and traumatised": Users' experiences of maternity care in the UK during the COVID-19 pandemic. Midwifery. 2021 Nov 1;102:103069.

15. McKinstry B et al. The use of telemonitoring in managing the COVID-19 pandemic: pilot implementation study. JMIR formative research. 2021 Sep 27;5(9):e20131.

16. Das R. Women's experiences of maternity and perinatal mental health services during the first Covid-19 lockdown. Journal of Health Visiting. 2021 Jul 2;9(7):297-303.

17. Altman MR et al. Where the system failed: the COVID-19 pandemic's impact on pregnancy and birth care. Global Qualitative Nursing Research. 2021 Mar;8:23333936211006397.

18. Horsch A et al. Moral and mental health challenges faced by maternity staff during the COVID-19 pandemic. Psychological Trauma. 2020 Aug;12(S1):S141.

19. Adams C. Pregnancy and birth in the United States during the COVID-19 pandemic: The views of doulas. Birth. 2022 Mar;49(1):116-22.

20. Vasilevski V et al. Receiving maternity care during the COVID-19 pandemic: Experiences of women's partners and support persons. Women and Birth. 2022 May 1;35(3):298-306.

21. González-Timoneda A et al. Experiences and attitudes of midwives during the birth of a pregnant woman with COVID-19 infection: A qualitative study. Women and birth. 2021 Sep 1;34(5):465-72.

22. Asefa A et al. The impact of COVID-19 on the provision of respectful maternity care: findings from a global survey of health workers. Women and Birth. 2021 Sep 10.

23. Heggeness ML. Estimating the immediate impact of the COVID-19 shock on parental attachment to the labor market and the double bind of mothers. Review of Economics of the Household. 2020 Dec;18(4):1053-78.

Chapter 7: Why we carry on

1. McAra-Couper J et al. Partnership and reciprocity with women sustain Lead Maternity Carer midwives in practice. New Zealand College of Midwives Journal. 2014 Jun 1;49.

2. Medland J et al. Fostering psychosocial wellness in oncology nurses: addressing burnout and social support in the workplace. InOncology nursing forum 2004 Jan 1 (Vol. 31, No. 1).

3. Warmelink J et al. An explorative study of factors contributing to the job satisfaction of primary care midwives. Midwifery. 2015 1;31(4):482-8.

4. Rizvi R et al. Facets of career satisfaction for women physicians in the United States: a systematic review. Women & health. 2012 May 1;52(4):403-21.

5. Freeney Y, Fellenz MR. Work engagement as a key driver of quality of care: a study with midwives. Journal of Health Organization and Management. 2013 Jun 14.

6. Muckaden MA, Pandya SS. Motivation of volunteers to work in palliative care setting: a qualitative study. Indian Journal of Palliative Care. 2016 Jul;22(3):348.

7. Brown A, Shenker N. Receiving Screened Donor Human Milk for Their Infant Supports Parental Wellbeing: a Mixed-methods Study. BMC pregnancy and childbirth, 2022.

8. Masten AS, Gewirtz AH. Resilience in development: The importance of early childhood. Encyclopaedia of early childhood. 2006.

9. Matheson C et al Resilience of primary healthcare professionals working in challenging environments: a focus group study. British Journal of General Practice. 2016 Jul 1;66(648):e507-15.

10. Leap N et al. Relationships the glue that holds it all together. In Sustainability, midwifery, and birth. 2011:61-74.

11. Sandall, J. (1997) 'Midwives' burnout and continuity of care', *British Journal of Midwifery*, 5, 2: 106–11.

12. Duffield C et al. Nursing unit managers, staff retention and the work environment. Journal of clinical nursing. 201120(1-2):23-33.

13. Hunter B et al. Midwives in the UK: Levels of burnout, depression, anxiety, stress & associated predictors. *Midwifery*, 2019, 79.

14. Edmondson MC, Walker SB. Working in caseload midwifery care: The experience of midwives working in a birth centre in North Queensland. Women and Birth. 2014 Mar 1;27(1):31-6.

15. Mollart, L., Skinner, V.M., Newing, C. and Foureur, M., 2013. Factors that may influence midwives work-related stress and burnout. *Women and birth*, 26(1), pp.26-32.

Chapter 8: Tools for support

1. Mezey G et al. Midwives' perceptions and experiences of routine enquiry for domestic violence. BJOG. 2003 Aug 1;110(8):744-52.

2. Van Lith T. Art therapy in mental health: A systematic review of approaches and practices. The Arts in Psychotherapy, 2016, 47, 9-22.

3. O'Keefe EL, O'Keefe JH, Lavie CJ. Exercise counteracts the cardiotoxicity of psychosocial stress. InMayo Clinic Proceedings 2019 Sep 1 (Vol. 94, No. 9, pp. 1852-1864). Elsevier.

4. Masterton W et al. Greenspace interventions for mental health in clinical and non-clinical populations: What works, for whom, and in what circumstances?. Health & Place. 2020 Jul 1;64:102338.

5. Wendelboe-Nelson C et al. A scoping review mapping research on green space and associated mental health benefits. IJERPH. 2019 Jan;16(12):2081.

6. Huttunen P, Kokko L, Ylijukuri V. Winter swimming improves general well-being. International Journal of Circumpolar Health. 2004 Jun 1;63(2):140-4.

7. Field T. Massage therapy research review. Complementary therapies in clinical practice. 2016 Aug 1;24:19-31.

8. Song H et al. Effect of self-administered foot reflexology for symptom management in healthy persons: systematic review & meta analysis. Complementary therapies in medicine. 2015 1:79-89.

9. Hilton L et al. Meditation for posttraumatic stress: Systematic review and meta-analysis. Psychological Trauma: Theory, Research, Practice, and Policy. 2017 Jul;9(4):453.
10. Pascoe MC et al. Mindfulness mediates the physiological markers of stress: systematic review and meta-analysis. Journal of psychiatric research. 2017 Dec 1;95:156-78.
11. Brown B. Daring greatly: How the Courage to Be Vulnerable Transforms the Way We Live, Love, Parent, and Lead. 2018. Penguin books.
12. https://www.youtube.com/watch?v=8-JXOnFOXQk
13. https://www.goodreads.com/quotes/7-it-is-not-the-critic-who-counts-not-the-man
14. https://www.acas.org.uk/discrimination-bullying-and-harassment
15. https://www.rcog.org.uk/careers-and-training/starting-your-og-career/workforce/improving-workplace-behaviours/workplace-behaviour-toolkit/
16. www.bma.org.uk/advice-and-support/your-wellbeing/self-help-questionnaires/worried-you-may-be-burning-out .
17. www.nhs.uk/every-mind-matters/mental-health-issues/stress/ .

Chapter 9: A manifesto for change

1. Kramer MS, Kakuma R. The optimal duration of exclusive breastfeeding. Protecting infants through human milk. 2004:63-77.
2. Brown A, Chucha S, Trickey H. Becoming breastfeeding friendly in Wales: Recommendations for scaling up breastfeeding support. Maternal & Child Nutrition. 2022 Apr 11:e13355.
3. Buccini G et al. How does "Becoming Breastfeeding Friendly" work? A programme impact pathways analysis. MCN, 2019, 15(3), e12766.
4. Moukarzel S et al. Breastfeeding promotion on Twitter: A social network and content analysis approach. Maternal & child nutrition, 2020 16(4), e13053.
5. Trickey H et al. A realist review of one-to-one breastfeeding peer support experiments conducted in developed country settings. MCN, 2018, 14(1), e12559.
6. Grant A et al. Availability of breastfeeding peer support in the United Kingdom: A cross-sectional study. MCN, 2018, 14(1), e12476.
7. Pérez-Escamilla R et al. Scaling up of breastfeeding promotion programs in low-and middle-income countries: the "breastfeeding gear" model. Advances in nutrition, 2012, 3(6), 790-800.
8. Brown, A. (2017). Breastfeeding as a public health responsibility: A review of the evidence. JHND, 30(6), 759-770.
9. Masters R et al Return on investment of public health interventions: a systematic review. Epidemiol Community Health, 2017, 71, 827-834.
10. McFadden A et al. Support for healthy breastfeeding mothers with healthy term babies. Cochrane Database of Systematic Reviews. 2017(2).
11. Brown A. Breastfeeding Uncovered: Who really decides how we feed our babies? 2021. Second edition. Pinter & Martin Ltd.

12. https://ukbreastfeeding.org/wbtiuk2016/
13. Hanson, M & Gluckman, P. Developmental origins of health and disease–global public health implications. *Best practice & research Clinical obstetrics & gynaecology*, 2015, 29(1), 24-31.
14. Azad M. et al (2021). Breastfeeding and the origins of health: interdisciplinary perspectives and priorities. *MCN*, 2021,17, e13109.
15. Kass, N. E. (2001). An ethics framework for public health. *American journal of public health*, 91(11), 1776-1782.
16. Hastings G et al. Selling second best: how infant formula marketing works. Globalization and Health. 2020 Dec;16(1):1-2.
17. Brown A et al. Marketing of infant milk in the UK: what do parents see and believe? First Steps Nutrition Trust: London. 2020
18. Munblit D, Crawley H, Hyde R, Boyle RJ. Health and nutrition claims for infant formula are poorly substantiated and potentially harmful. bmj. 2020 May 6;369.
19. Pyles T et al. (2021). Breastfeeding sisters that are receiving support: Community-based peer support program created for and by women of color. *Breastfeeding Medicine*, 2021,16(2), 165– 170.
20. Rutter PM, Jones W. Enquiry analysis and user opinion of the Drugs in Breastmilk Helpline: a prospective study. International breastfeeding journal. 2012 May;7(1):6
21. Amir LH. Medicines for breastfeeding women: risky business. Breastfeeding: Methods, Benefits to the Infant and Mother and Difficulties. 2010:129-41
22. Anderson PO et al. Adverse drug reactions in breastfed infants: less than imagined. Clin Pediatr (Phila) 2003;42(4):325-40.
23. Brodribb W et al: Attitudes to infant feeding decision-making–a mixed-methods study of Australian medical students and GP registrars. Breastfeed Rev. 2010, 18 (1): 5-13.
24. Amir LH et al. Avoiding risk at what cost? Putting use of medicines for breastfeeding women into perspective. International breastfeeding journal. 2012 Dec;7(1):14
25. https://breastfeedingnetwork.org.uk/wp-content/pdfs/BfN%20Final%20report%20.pdf

Index